MAKING FACES

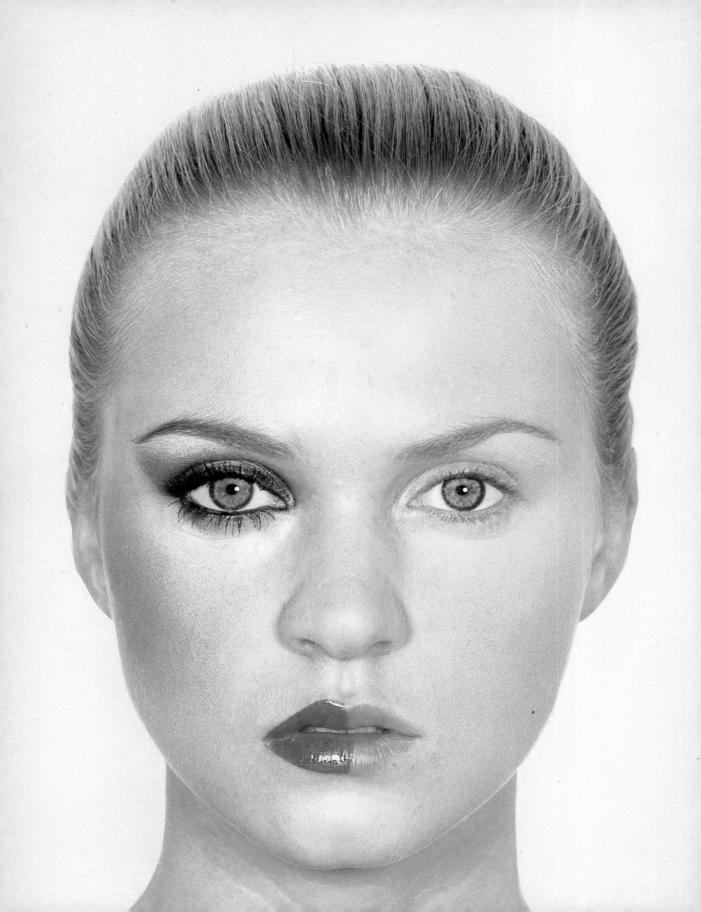

Joan Price & Pat Booth

MAKING FACES

Name _PAUL KNOWLES_

Unit/Module _ARTS BLOCK_

Subject _GRAPHICS_

Option Group/Year _ROOM A3_

Academic Year 201   201

Michael Joseph
London

CONTENTS

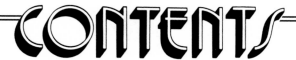

CONTENTS

foundation and colour build-up – the use of colour to emphasize changing focal points of the face – current balance between eyes and mouth – the coordination of make-up colours and clothes – effect of lighting

To MICHAEL
without whom there would be
no Face Places and no Making Faces

First published in Great Britain by Michael Joseph Limited, 44 Bedford Square, London WC1   1980
© 1980 by Joan Price and Pat Booth
ISBN 0 7181 1878 2
Designed by Penny Mills
Printed and bound by New Interlitho Spa, Milan, Italy

ATTITUDES TO FACE

It has always seemed quite natural to me that every woman should want to look her best. I have never been one to believe that in the next world I shall do penance for every lipstick I have ever bought. But over the years I have become increasingly aware that my attitude is far from being universally held.

Being neither a moralist nor over-intellectual, I have never worried overmuch about the pros and cons of wearing make-up. To me it is just as unnatural not to want to look one's best as other women may think it unnatural to look anything other than exactly how they were born.

The basic purpose of make-up today is to do what it has done throughout history. To glamorize women's looks. That is not to say that it has not taken on subsidiary roles. For instance, many women with bad skins caused by acne or with redness due to over-exposure to the sun have found make-up invaluable in helping to hide their imperfections.

If you pause to think about make-up, you will realize that most developed civilizations have used it extensively, although in modern society a number of extremes are apparent which need a sociologist to understand and interpret. In the last sixty years we have fluctuated between the made-up look and the natural look.

When we are in a period when the made-up look is fashionable, such as in the 1930s and 1940s, a woman who wishes to be in fashion will have no choice but to wear make-up. When a more natural look is in vogue, as today, make-up still has an important role to play, however, accentuating one's good points and minimizing one's defects. It is possible that a young girl, especially if she is dark-haired, can get away with not wearing make-up, but once a woman has reached thirty, it is most unlikely that she is going to look her best without a little artificial aid. If she is fair, it is only by using make-up that she will lend her features any definition.

Psychologists in recent years have begun to take an interest in the whole question of looking one's best. If you are one of those people who worries

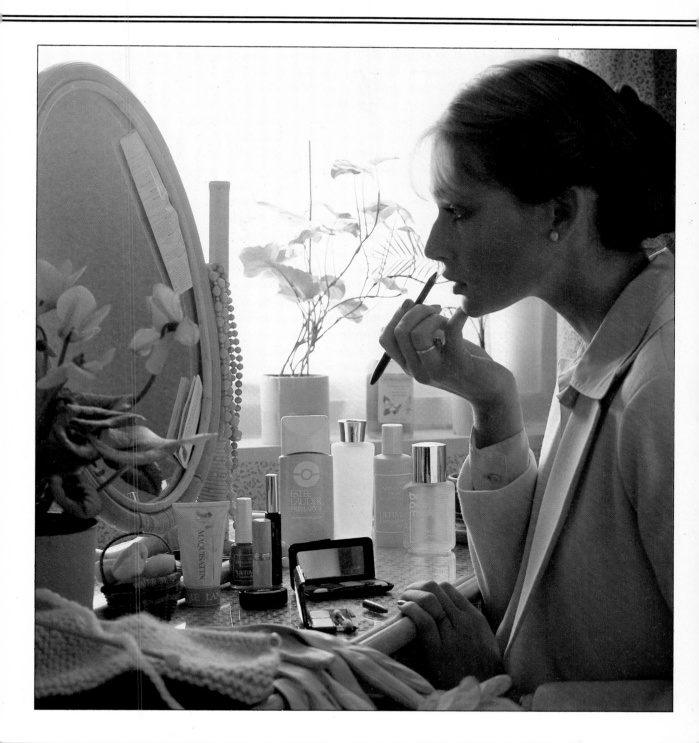

about spending too much time, trouble and money on looking good, here is some recent research which may reassure you.

In an article in *New Society* in November 1974, Ray Bull, a lecturer in Psychology at the North East London Polytechnic, discussed "the importance of being beautiful". He referred to an experiment carried out the previous year in the United States where it was found that the attractiveness of the defendant in a law case had a significant effect upon jurors' decisions about the length of sentence given. In this article he also mentioned two other pieces of research. Kaven Dim of Toronto University concluded that "good-looking people are seen as possessing more socially desirable traits and as having more future potential for happiness and success than unattractive individuals". Psychologist Arthur Miller found that undergraduates rated the attractive as "more curious, complex, perceptive, academic, restless, confident, assertive, happy, active, amiable, humorous, pleasure-seeking, outspoken and flexible than the unattractive individuals".

In another research test, attractiveness ratings were found to be significantly higher for women wearing make-up; and it was found that make-up had a considerable effect on the way people were perceived by others. It was particularly interesting to note that although the observers were asked what they thought had influenced their impressions, none in fact thought to mention make-up. In another test attractive people were seen as "more intelligent, honest, stable and friendly". I have quoted these research experiments at some length because I feel that some people tend to have quite strongly ingrained attitudes of hostility towards the use of make-up, without ever considering its many advantages and the reasons why women wear it. What has emerged from recent research is that attractiveness is one of the major dimensions of interpersonal perception.

Intuitively women in all civilizations have known this. There has hardly been a developed civilization in which make-up has not been used; indeed, it could be said that make-up has been synonymous with the highest points of the world's civilization.

All the early civilizations which derived from the Euphrates Valley used make-up extensively. The Egyptians are the most obvious example of a civilization which developed their extremely artificial looks to a fine art; the use of kohl and mascara can certainly be traced back to them. The frescoes at Knossos show us the extent to which eye make-up was used by the Minoan civilization in Crete, influenced perhaps by their Egyptian trading partners. Art at Pompeii indicates both the amount of time that the Romans spent at their toilette and the amount of make-up they used. As for the

Byzantians, those superb mosaics in the Church of St Vitale at Ravenna reveal clearly that the remarkable Empress Theodora used cosmetics to produce a look which by any standards would be considered artificial and made-up

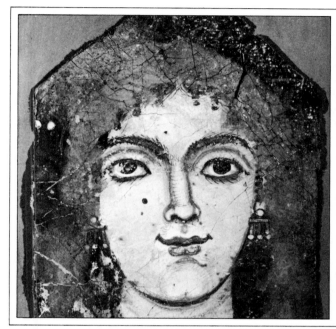

The extensive use of kohl and mascara in eye make-up, as portrayed by this young girl in Roman Egypt during the fourth century AD, can be traced back to the Ancient Egyptians.

The Chinese, who have had the longest and most continuous civilization, spent considerable time and trouble on their appearance with quite extraordinary preferences. For instance, as great admirers of small feet, they bound their female children's feet at birth, so that they would always remain small and neat. It was the Chinese, too, who developed excessively long nails – presumably as proof that one was rich and prosperous enough not to have to do anything as demeaning as manual work.

The most striking feature which becomes apparent in reviewing attitudes to make-up over thousands of years is that it is Judaism, with its basic conception of Eve leading Adam to his downfall, which has been most vehemently opposed to the idea of women beautifying themselves. The endless stories in the Bible of women leading men astray, of harlots, painted faces and Jezebels, are all ones which the early Christian Church absorbed and they have influenced Western thought ever since.

Apart from this though, I can see little evidence that before the spread of Christianity other civilizations had had reservations about the pleasure of looking one's best and using make-up. There is no denying that the Church's attitude has caused considerable swings of the pendulum and dichotomies since the fall of the Roman Empire. Oddly enough, it seemed to have less effect on the Byzantine Empire, which in some historians' view was the most truly Christian of all empires, but where luxury, exotic appearance and the lavish use of cosmetics were strongly favoured. Perhaps this was due to its proximity to the ways of the East.

The paradox crops up continually in the Middle Ages. As Europe emerged from its dark years, the Church dominated men's minds almost completely. The Crusaders, however, brought back to Europe many of the ideas and luxuries which they had encountered in the Middle East. In her novel *The World is Not Enough*, Zoe Oldenbourg writes, "he learned that there were women who rubbed their teeth with herbs to make them bright, who perfumed their hair with Arabian essences, who washed their faces and bodies in milk and oil and wore knots of sweet-smelling herbs between their breasts. Edith twined threads of gold and strings of pearls into her hair, she wore embroidered shifts of white silk, she spent hours whitening her hands and arranging her hair."

In her fascinating book on the fourteenth century, *A Distant Mirror*, Barbara Tuchman gives us a marvellous picture of man's constant pull between the Church's disapproval and the allurement of female beauty. She writes, "No female iniquity was more severely condemned than the habit of plucking eyebrows and the hairline to heighten the forehead. For some reason a particular immorality was attached to it, perhaps because it altered God's arrangements. Demons in purgatory were said to punish the practice by sticking 'hot burning awls and needles' into every hole from which a hair had been plucked."

After the Protestant Reformation, this attitude gained momentum. Philip Stubbes in his famous polemic against the new, pleasurable or man-made habits of the Elizabethan age wrote, "The women of Anglia colour their faces with certain oyles, liquors, unguents and waters made to that end, whereby they think their beautie is greatly desired: but who seeth not that their soules are thereby deformed. . . ."

The two most notable fashions were the wearing of patches, that is little black beauty spots which showed off the whiteness of the skin, and shaving the hair together with plucking the eyebrows to achieve the fashionable high forehead.

The Puritan Revolution did not succeed in changing attitudes as

In the Middle Ages, no female vanity was more severely condemned than the fashion of plucking the eyebrows and the hairline to heighten the forehead.

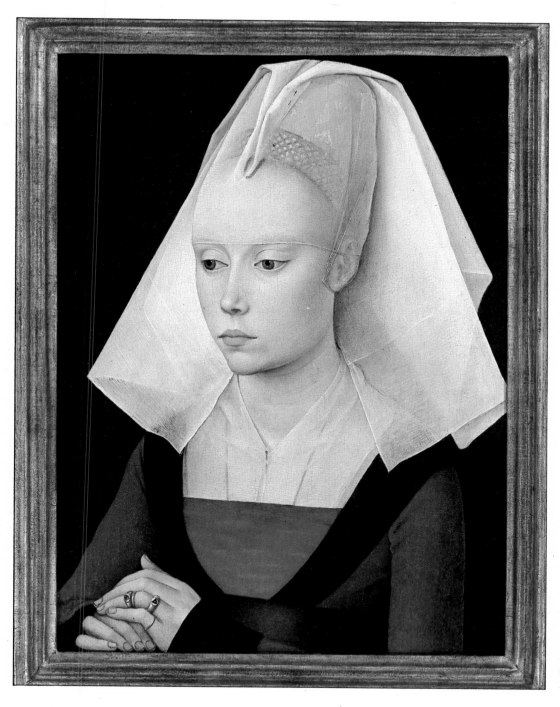

Portrait of a
Lady by R. van
der Weyden,
*National
Portrait Gallery
London.*

drastically as might have been expected. Nevertheless, in 1653, in a book entitled *The Loathsomness of Long Haire*, Thomas Hull, a clergyman, still found it necessary to add "a word concerning the vanities and exorbitances of many women, in painting, patching, spotting and blotting themselves".

From the Restoration and throughout the eighteenth century, there was a much more relaxed attitude to make-up and beauty, but in the nineteenth century the tide turned again with the coming of the Victorian age.

The excesses of the Regency caused the Victorians to rebel against the artificiality of a period when some women actually poisoned themselves with toxic concoctions of mercury, lime and even carbolic acid: they used these mixtures to enamel their faces to such an extent that some of them were afraid to smile lest they crack their perfect porcelain finish. So strong was the Victorian reaction that it became fashionable to wear no make-up, and ugliness was seen almost as a moral virtue.

I believe that there is a need to stress that the resurgence of make-up in the twentieth century marks the revival of attitudes held prior to the nineteenth century. In fact it was the nineteenth century with its "back to nature" principle which was unique, rather than the twentieth with its use of cosmetics. The essential difference in this century from all previous ones is that make-up is now applied by all classes of society, rather than being primarily the preserve of royal courts and the leisured classes.

It is difficult to pinpoint any single reason: there are many involved. Rising standards of living, mass media and communications for advertising and promotion, far greater availability and choice of products have all led to the wider use of make-up; and as I discuss in a later chapter, perhaps the greatest persuader of all was the cinema in the twenties, thirties and fifties, setting a standard for the ideal look which became the aim of every woman.

With the increasing use of cosmetics and the infinitely broader scope of fashion, we have seen in the last twenty years a new phenomenon: new fashions started by the young and then taken up by older members of society, such as the no lipstick look, which was started by the young as a reaction to the crimson red lips of their mothers, and the wearing of more casual clothes like jeans.

I still find, however, that the disapprobation of the past as regards make-up has left its mark in this country perhaps more than in any other. Maybe it is because I am English and live in this country and am more aware of Englishmen and their inhibitions, but it really does seem that the French and Italians have a more relaxed attitude to beautiful women than the English.

I cannot believe that there is any other country in the world where the

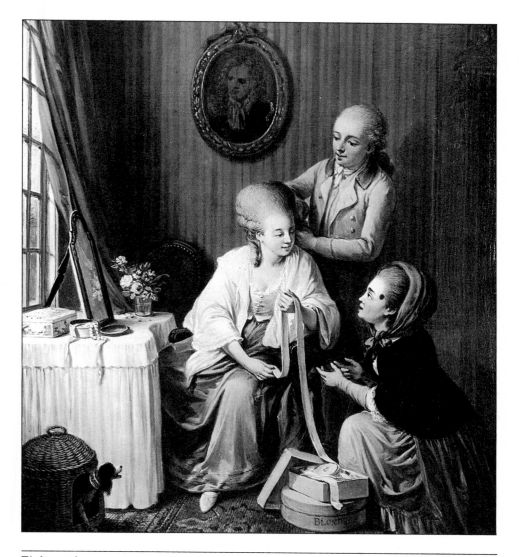

Eighteenth-century excesses included elaborate coiffures and the liberal application of black beauty spots.

following conversation, which took place in my shop in Cadogan Street, could have occurred:

"Good lord, Jane – what are you doing here!" (Laughter.)

"I say, don't tell George, he'd die laughing to think of me in a beauty shop." (More laughter.)

"Darling, don't be silly, if Henry knew I'd been having my face done he'd think I'd gone crazy. He'd say, 'Darling, they couldn't do much with your face old girl! – perhaps he's right." (Peals of laughter.)

In France, George and Henry would assume that their wives went to a beauty shop at least once a week, and would perhaps worry if they did not.

Of course, to a large extent our ideas are formed and influenced by our parents: in my experience this is nowhere more apparent than in the case of men's attitudes to make-up. So much seems to depend on what their mothers did. This is unfortunate in that most of us currently use much more make-up than was used, say, thirty or forty years ago, even if we do apply it more subtly.

I am always amused when I meet a man for the first time and he asks me what I do. When I say "I run beauty shops," I frequently get interesting comments and certainly quite different from those I would get if I said I ran a book shop: somehow the latter would appear to him safer, more normal and less aggressive. I will never forget, when I had just opened my shop, talking to a colleague of my husband's who was a director of a large advertising agency; he asked if I did not feel worried starting a business which encouraged women to spend lots of money on make-up. Why, I asked, was it any worse than spending money on food or drink? He felt it was: "You shouldn't encourage women to spend money on something like make-up, which encourages them to be something they aren't." He felt it was a form of cheating – and this from an advertising man!

Another man I know, an actor no less, told me he approved of make-up, but found the idea of kissing a woman's eyes when she was wearing eye-shadow and mascara a worrying one.

Men do like pretty and attractive girls, but it does seem to me that they like to feel that they were born that way. A little lipstick is all right, but more is regarded as a deception.

There may also be a tendency on the part of some Englishmen to see wives as a combination of a charming mother, sister, and housekeeper: someone maternal, friendly and efficient. In making themselves look more beautiful women are not fulfilling the wifely function which they are meant to aspire to. Beauty is irrelevant to this role. So in a typically English way, when embarrassed by a subject, we make it a "hoot": hence George and Henry. Surrounded by such attitudes it takes a determined woman to fight them.

Money spent on beauty becomes a low priority. My observation is that an Englishwoman's priorities in spending her money are, first her children, then the house, the garden, and even the dog, and last herself. On the Continent the priority will be herself first of all, then the others in almost reverse order.

If you think I am exaggerating let me quote the top executive of a leading American company: she once told me that England is the only country where in department stores women will put down half their cosmetic purchases on the account and pay for the other half themselves.

Nevertheless, many women's lack of confidence in their ability to select the right make-up is frequently reflected in their purchase of high price cosmetics. Estée Lauder has always understood that a high price gives confidence and is seen as an endorsement of quality: she has never been afraid of pricing her products at the top of the market.

When I started the Face Place twelve years ago, I thought that it was going to be the teenage to twenty-four-year-old single girls who would be the backbone of the business. In fact, I could not have been more wrong. These girls are the very people who do not need help. Many of them work in offices, or share flats with other girls. They talk about make-up, discuss what products and brands they use, they buy their cosmetics at Boots: they

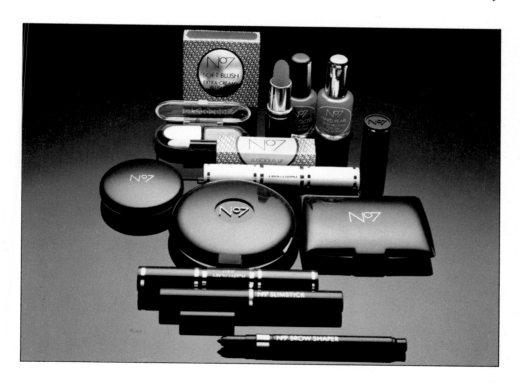

buy the less expensive brands because they are confident of their choice and because the price of these cosmetics allows for the impulse or occasional wrong buy.

In recent years Boots has done a lot to help the buying of cosmetics. In the last ten years they have realized what an important part cosmetic sales play in their overall operation. Not only have they carried out an extremely professional job in revamping their No. 7 range, but they also offer an extremely wide range of cosmetics from the expensive to cheaper brands. It is not surprising that they sell about one in three of all cosmetics sold in this country.

It is as a girl grows older that she may lose touch with make-up trends and habits. If she gets married and has children, talk about babies and domestic matters takes over from the more light-hearted and frivolous chat of unattached girls discussing fashion trends, the latest lipstick colour or where to get their hair cut. Or if she is a career girl, it may be that the increasing interest in her job means that she discusses make-up less. Either way, gradually and imperceptibly she falls behind, using the same colours as she did five years ago. And then she says to a friend in the same position as herself, who has decided she wants to do something to improve her looks, "I had a lovely time yesterday, I tried on a new face."

It is just these women who are the supporters of the Face Place. They want advice and help on how to bring their faces up-to-date; perhaps because they are going to a smart party, or just because they feel it is time they did something different.

A powerful influence on middle-aged women wanting advice are their teenage daughters. A mother seeing her sixteen-year-old daughter building up her eye colour will be quite surprised at the time and trouble that her daughter takes. Then she sees the effect and thinks it could be attractive; she realizes then how out of fashion she is and decides that something must be done.

Fashions and trends in make-up do change just as they do in clothes. But in some ways it is more difficult to appreciate this. Make-up fashions change more slowly and less obviously than clothes and they are written about less. But if you look at pictures in fashion magazines of, say, ten years ago, you will see what I mean. For instance, to wear Cleopatra eyes today will date you every bit as much as wearing a mini-skirt. How your face looks really is important. In case you feel that since beauty is my business I am biased, let me quote two leading fashion experts. Thea Porter, the well-known designer who was in the forefront of the introduction of the kaftan and exotic Eastern evening dresses, said a few years ago, "Get the face right and you can wear anything." And Prudence Glynn, the authoritative fashion editor of *The Times*, has said, "Nothing dates you more than an out-of-date face."

It is, I think, one of the problems of the beauty business generally that it tends to restrict its appeal to the existing heavy users of make-up who buy plenty of cosmetics. Their method of selling in stores is almost completely geared to an existing market, and instead of trying to widen this market many of the leading brands seem content to chase each other's customers, with offers like a free gift tied to another product, or as the trade calls it, "free gift with purchase". So much of cosmetic advertising seems to be directed at the already converted. Almost the only exception is that carried out by the manufacturers of the young ranges, who mainly advertise in the teenage magazines. These manufacturers, perhaps because they are not so strongly represented in the stores and especially because they are appealing to a growing-up market, seem much more aware of the need to educate their public to their products. However, the general tendency of exclusivity, together with the fact that more and more new products are introduced each year, means that a wedge is gradually being driven between "those in the know" and "those outside the magic circle".

It is a major problem for many women to find a way into this magic circle, and I am particularly aware how difficult it is for women over thirty who do not use, or have never used, a lot of make-up. When training new girls in my shop I say to them, "Think of our customers as if they were coming into a hardware shop to buy a half inch nail: whatever you do, don't send them away as so many hardware shops do, feeling that they know nothing about anything, and that it would have been much better if they had never come into this shop in the first place."

By encouraging their consultants to look too made-up and flawless, the manufacturers in my opinion help to perpetuate the problem. Many women, usually those "outside the magic circle", complain that so many of the store consultants scare them to death. They make comments like, "The girls in the stores look so grand that they make me feel dowdy." Whether it is entirely because of their appearance or because the customer feels trapped into buying more than she means to, the end result tends to be one of mistrust. Unfortunately this is usually on the part of the women who know least about make-up and are the least confident. Women experienced in buying cosmetics are seldom worried by this aspect of the beauty business.

At the other extreme are the many chemists who sell cosmetics and are unable to offer the customer expert advice. Incidentally have you ever stopped to wonder why cosmetics should be sold in chemists at all? After all, the chemist and his assistants are not experts in the latest colours, or for that matter not usually particularly versed in how to apply the latest products such as blushers or shapers. The truth, of course, is that in the twenties and thirties when it was considered daring and possibly dangerous to put paint on to one's face, the fact that cosmetics were sold by trained ethical pharmacists made them seem clinically acceptable. I am inclined to the view that the average chemist is not the ideal outlet for selling cosmetics, since most of us have overcome the feeling that cosmetics may be dangerous for our skin. Again in the days when cosmetics were confined mainly to lipstick and powder, there were no problems in the chemist stocking and selling these products. But today, when there may be two dozen colours in a lipstick range alone, ten in a foundation, five shades in blusher and sixteen shades in eyeshadow, it needs a degree of expertise in make-up rather than in pharmacy to stock a shop selling cosmetics.

No chapter on attitudes to beauty would be complete without a word on the controversial subject of beauty without cruelty, or to put it more accurately, the testing of cosmetics on animals. Some of my clients even produce a "black list" of manufacturers whose products are to be avoided because they are supposed to carry out animal testing in laboratories.

My argument may not be acceptable to everyone, but in fact the more you know about cosmetics the more I think you will agree with me. The problem about "beauty without cruelty" is that it is an emotive idea. There is no such thing as a good commercial product that is not dependent for some of its ingredients on research done and tested on animals by some of the major manufacturers many years ago for the basic raw materials used nowadays by all manufacturers. This applies to commercially-produced herbal creams and lotions as well. However basic and natural the product ingredients are, you need, as in packaged foods, stabilizers and preservatives, if the mixtures are not to go rancid and quickly lose their consistency. It is these stabilizers and preservatives which can be the cause of skin irritants unless they have been extensively tested, and I am afraid that there is no alternative that I know of to animal testing. Truthfully, if you are against animal testing you would be better to wear no make-up or skin-care products at all, other than those short-lived products you can make yourself.

It is one of the purposes of this book that it should help you to understand that the world of beauty is like any other world: an analogy with cooking helps to make the point. Until you start cooking it all seems a mystery, but once you understand the general principles you become more confident and begin to enjoy it. I assure you that beauty is the same. Please do not think that because it is something you know little about it has to remain a mystery for ever. Of course, as with cooking, a little flair helps, but it is knowing the ground rules which really makes the difference. Do not be put off by some of the more fantastic claims, exotic names and the generally sophisticated aura in which the products are sold. A word of encouragement if you know little about it and feel lost: there are a lot of other women around like you. You are not unique, at least in this respect. What is sad is that so many women feel that the world of beauty is closed to them – it is not.

Unfortunately, I often think that this attitude is encouraged by the style in which so many glossy magazine articles are written, as well as by that which many of the cosmetic houses' consultants adopt in department stores. Although magazines can to some extent be helpful sources for ideas and guidance about beauty, they often suffer from the fact that many editors know less about beauty than they would care to admit, and so are happy to see articles which make a mystique out of beauty.

Having worked for over twenty years on magazines, I have always been puzzled by the fact that most editors are perfectly happy to have relatively down-to-earth and factual articles on, say, cooking, but once they come to beauty they seem to expect the language to become flowery, full of adjectives, and to my mind altogether less comprehensible. Perhaps editors feel that as beauty is a subject they do not understand themselves, it must be complicated; but I have never appreciated why they should think that their readers are in a more knowledgeable position than they are. Or could it be that beauty articles are basically a product of the twenties and thirties and therefore have acquired and retained a style suitable to a more leisured and pampered readership, whereas cookery writing, which has its roots in the forties and fifties, has a much more straightforward tradition? Or perhaps it is that art directors on magazines see their opportunity to do something really creative, and so the picture which illustrates the article is used for its visual effect rather than to make a point. Whatever the reason, it helps to create this unfortunate attitude of beauty being an exclusive world, an in-world to which you need a special passport.

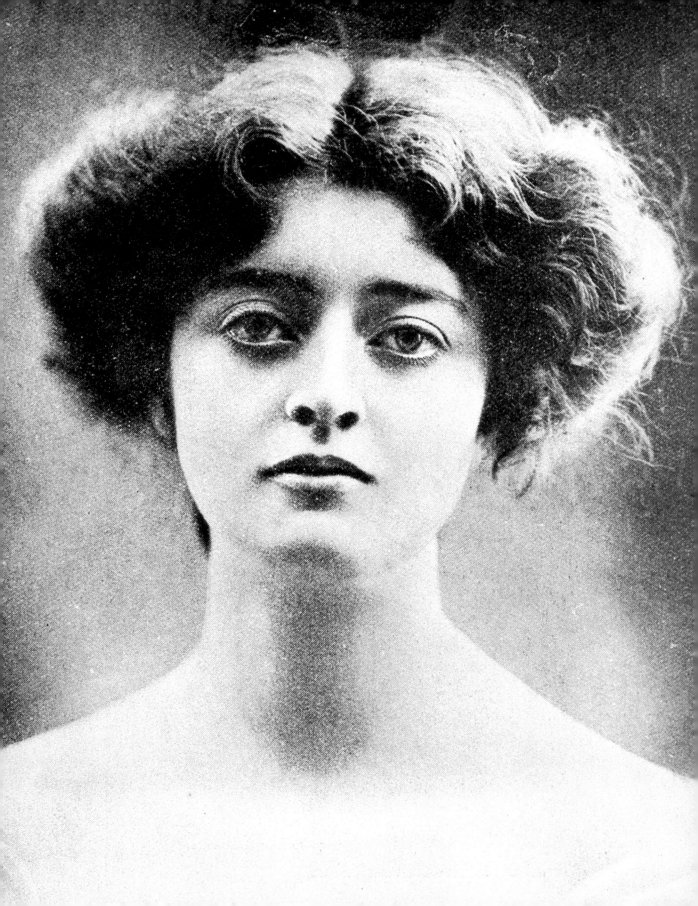

CHANGING FACE OF FASHION

In the course of the twentieth century it is impossible to stress just how dramatic an effect the rise of the communication media, in particular the cinema and glossy magazines, has had on setting new ideals of beauty and changing established principles. In glamorous film stars and models, there were examples of perfection which became every woman's aim. Another source of inspiration has been the cosmetic innovators: turning a clever new idea into a reality requires vision and courage, but many such individuals have come to dominate the industry and so influence your looks.

Make-up as we know it today really started after the First World War. Until then, it had consisted generally of a few discreet aids, such as coloured powder and rouge. Few men realized that women were wearing any make-up. The idea that make-up should look provocative and be seen to be artificial came with the twenties. It is difficult to assess exactly what caused this new outlook, but it must have been a combination of circumstances.

Attitudes had changed dramatically after the First World War: women had taken on jobs, formerly done by men; in Britain they received the vote; they felt and became more liberated. Make-up became one expression of these new trends.

With this general liberation we find that skirts became shorter for the first time at the beginning of the twenties, and women were eager to copy Coco Chanel's short bobbed hair, which made the Eton crop so fashionable. It is difficult for us, so used every day to seeing the widest array of fashion imaginable, to realize quite what a revolution it was for our grandmothers to raise their skirts and cut off their hair. For as long as people could remember long hair had been everyone's ambition and normal young girls aimed to grow their hair long enough to be able to sit on it.

Before the emancipation of women, make-up was subtle rather than provocative, and consisted of a few discreet aids such as powder, powder rouge and a touch of tinted cream rouge on the lips.

Harriet Hubbard Ayer

Like many other society ladies in the late nineteenth century, Mrs Hubbard Ayer of Chicago collected her own beauty recipes for the creams and lotions she used on her face, in the same way that today we have our favourite recipes for cooking. When her rich industrialist husband lost all his money speculating, her marriage broke up and she moved to Paris where she went into business selling cosmetics.

She was the first person to understand that selling cosmetics was like selling clothes; if you wanted to sell your products they needed to be promoted, and the best way was by the personal recommendation of a well-known celebrity.

A naturally talented writer, she had a great instinct for recognizing trends. It seemed to her that women's attitudes to the use of face creams, and even tinted foundations, were changing, and products which were once shunned were coming into fashion.

Having written a promotional booklet for Ponds called ''A Woman's Birthright—How every woman may look her best'', she later used some testimonials from other

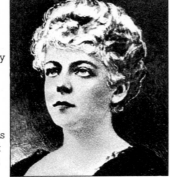

Harriet Hubbard Ayer, a forerunner of today's fashion.

women to promote her products. She claimed that one of her best selling creams was from a recipe used by the legendary beauty of Napoleonic France, Madame Récamier. In the 1880s, at the time of her most prolific writings, women were still divided into two groups; the few who painted their faces

and the many who didn't: of the former some admitted that they did, while many others pretended they didn't.

Harriet Hubbard Ayer was of course completely in favour of the use of cosmetics, particularly for what she described as ''hiding imperfections'' and ''delicately simulating womanly charms by using every aid known to cosmetic art''.

She deplored the male chauvinist attitudes which accused her of being a Jezebel, providing women with cosmetic artifice to use on their faces. She strongly

condemned men who disapproved of their wives even using a little toilet powder and yet succumbed to the charms of other painted and peroxided ladies.

Many of her cosmetics were forerunners of today's cosmetics: she pioneered tinted powder, which she called 'Velouté powder', and led the fashion for darkening the eyebrows with black and brown 'Ford Indian' which she named after the paint used by Indians; Baton au Raisin was a wine-coloured stick which she developed to give a warm red glow to the lips and was the forerunner of lipstick.

Her company still continues today, although it hasn't a presence in the United Kingdom. Now owned by a major international conglomerate it is flourishing in France.

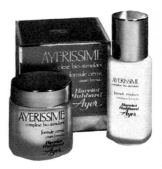

Elegant skin care products incorporating Bio Stimulenes for combating ageing skin and wrinkles.

Their resident visagiste, Olivier Echaudemaison is much in demand for make-up work with top photographers in many countries and he did the make-up for Norman Parkinson's pictures of Princess Anne at the time of her wedding.

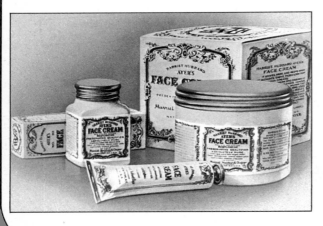

The packaging for one of Harriet Hubbard Ayer's early products, Face Cream which was sold in these attractively labelled pots and tubes and bought by beauties at the turn of the century

Suddenly the Eton crop changed everything: the face was revealed and make-up came into its own to ensure that what was seen looked at its best. For the first time the tips of the ears were shown, and gently rouged by those in the height of fashion. Even *Vogue* was a bit taken aback by the new fashions and in 1923 was complaining, "The painted faces that one sometimes meets (but more fortunately on the Continent) pass well enough when seen in repose, but in animation or at close range, their artificiality is painfully apparent."

Fashion for faces had arrived. The face was pale and powdery looking without a trace of natural shine. Vanishing cream on the nose held powder in place. One of the most popular of the early face powders was called Flesh, a peach-tinted confection which women applied with a swansdown handkerchief puff. The more adventurous leaders of fashion shined up their eyelids with Vaseline and plucked their eyebrows into a pin-thin crescent line, lengthened with

black eyebrow pencil. Lashes were darkened with black block mascara. Cream rouge was worn high on cheeks and even applied to newly exposed earlobes. Colourless lip gloss was a top seller, but by the mid-twenties lipstick colours such as vermilion and carmine red were beginning to be worn. These early lip colours contained plenty of indelible stain that was intended to make them kiss-proof.

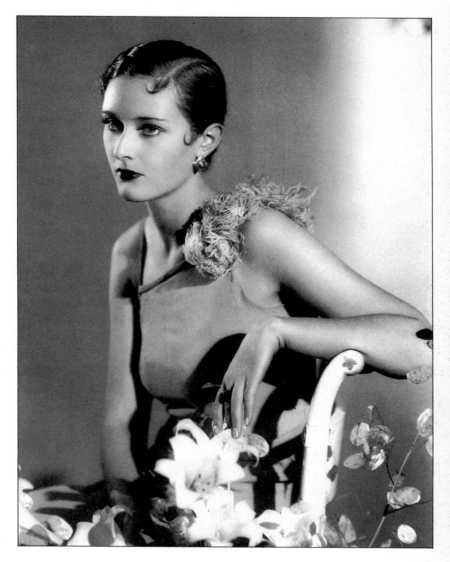

Twenties make-up and the
Eton Crop

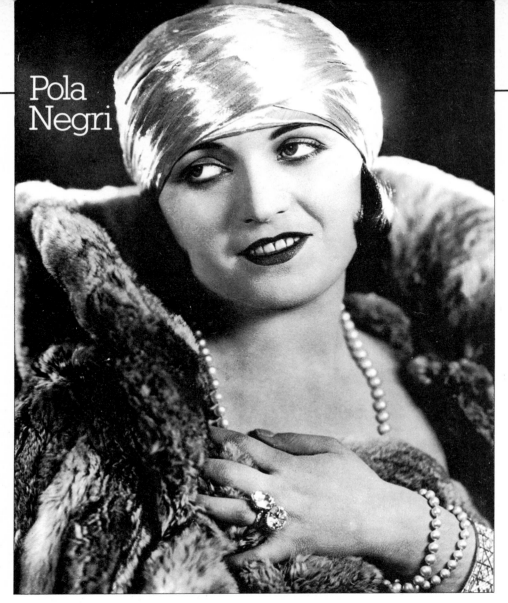

Pola Negri

In the meantime, the influence of the cinema, perhaps the greatest influence of all in looks, had begun to be felt. Stars of the silent screen such as Pola Negri, Theda Bara and Mary Pickford set new styles. Pola Negri and Theda Bara were prototypes for the "vamp" look, while Mary Pickford became everyone's idea of the perfect "sweetheart". To achieve these looks make-up experts were required. One of the first to move to Hollywood was Max Factor, a Polish stage make-up artist who had worked for the Moscow State Theatre.

The movies continued to dominate the make-up look into the thirties. Cinema stars like Greta Garbo, Marlene Dietrich and Joan Crawford became the trendsetters. Garbo's eyebrows were plucked into a thin line and

Helena Rubinstein

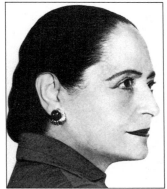

Helena Rubinstein

Like Harriet Hubbard Ayer, Madame Rubinstein understood the importance of celebrities and the early success of her skin-care creams and early make-up products was considerably accelerated by celebrities using them. Melba, the great Australian singer, was one of the first to become a follower when Helena Rubinstein arrived in Australia from Poland in the 1890s and opened her beauty salon in Melbourne. She brought with her to Australia many of the recipes for skin products developed by a chemist friend of her mother's, Dr Lykusky. In a country where everyone's skin was sunburnt, Helena Rubinstein's pale complexion was her best advertisement; it was constantly remarked on from the moment she arrived in Australia and helped to promote the excellence of her creams. With the help of Dr Lykusky, she formulated a whole range of products, including the first tinted powders which helped to hide the ravages of the sun, and gave a smooth even appearance to the skin.

Having established herself in Australia she decided to come to London where she rented Lord Salisbury's house in Grafton Street; she opened a very exclusive salon and again repeated her success with both products and treatments. Coming from a large family of girls, she employed her sisters as caretakers of her growing empire and wherever a salon was established, one of the Rubinstein sisters or a relation was left in charge.

As she says so appositely to today's cosmetic industry, when so many beauty manufacturing companies, including the one which bears her name, are being bought by international conglomerates, ''Both the cosmetic and fashion businesses, I have learned over the years, are best run as personal enterprises.''

She was the first to promote the idea of a ''day of beauty'', which meant including body treatments together with face and hair. In Paris with her second husband, Prince Artchil Gourielli, a White Russian, she ultimately launched a range of men's cosmetics. Today this seems a fairly obvious measure, but thirty years ago it was an adventurous step.

At the beginning of the First World War she went to America where she established yet another of her businesses in New York on the same pattern as she had before; once again she recognized the value of promotion, and since this was the era of the silent movies she helped to create the ''vamp'' look and the use of mascara featured by Theda Bara.

After the war she returned to Europe and opened a salon in the Faubourg St Honoré, in Paris. In the meantime, she had sold her American business to the well-known Wall Street bankers, Lehman Brothers, only to find that by the time of the Wall Street crash of 1929, the business had almost faded away. She was able, as she says in her autobiography, to ''buy back the controlling interest in the business for a fraction of what they had paid me!''

One of the main influences Helena Rubinstein had on the beauty business was to take and commercialize the aesthetic idea of skin care. Generally speaking, mid-Europeans have greasy and not very good skin. They understand the need to look after and treat their skin regularly. Helena Rubinstein took this concept, packaged it and promoted it, and became the biggest name in beauty; she probably made more money out of it than anyone has done before or since.

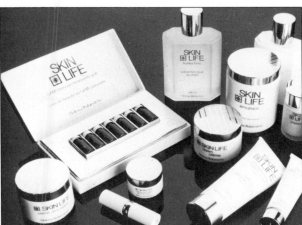

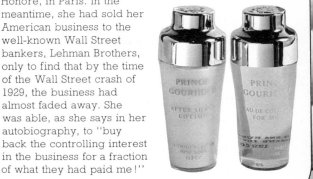

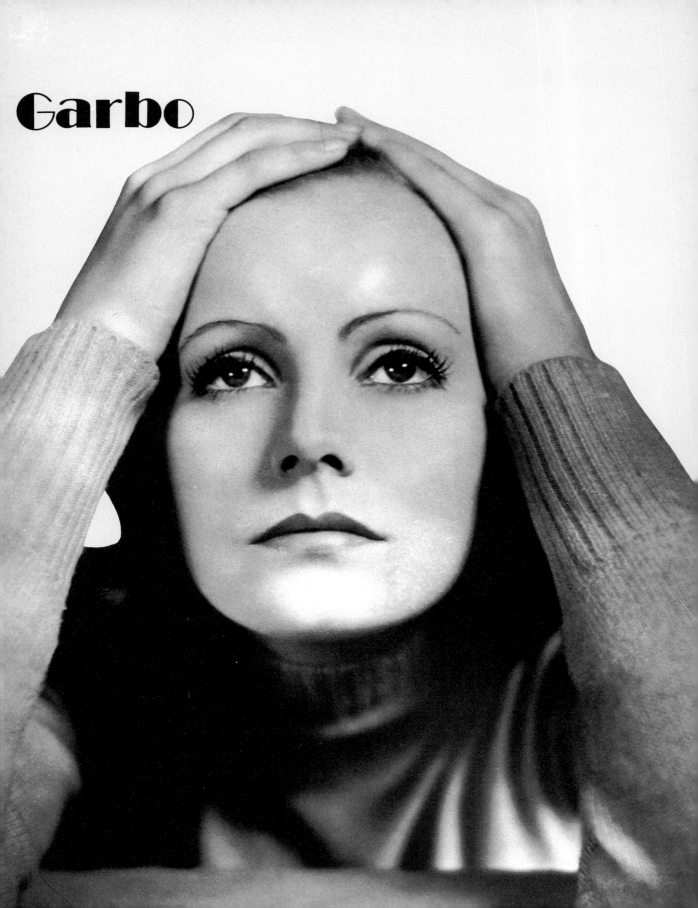

Garbo

lengthened with eyebrow pencil, and her trick of drawing a fine dark line on her eyelids was copied by women everywhere. Her longer hair was softly parted. The strident emancipated look was softening. But just as widely copied was the harsher look of Joan Crawford, with full red lips and heavily pencilled eyebrows.

New cosmetics were coming on to the market, as the manufacturers supplied products designed to create the effects which the stage make-up artists had achieved. This whole battery of new cosmetics included products such as cheek cream rouges in four shades, vermilion, flame, carmine and crimson, which were matched to the firmly established bright red lipsticks. Coloured eyeshadows were already being introduced, and were mainly used to enhance eyes, coming in green, blue and turquoise shades. Because they were in soft cream form it was necessary to make up eyelids with foundation and powder before using them, so that the soft cream colours did not melt. Charles Revson, introducing the dramatic idea of matching nail varnish to lipstick, became a major force in the cosmetic world overnight.

Photographs had begun to be used instead of fashion drawings to illustrate the new clothes in the glossy magazines. Models became a new influence on looks. Suddenly it was acceptable to be photographed for a glossy magazine, and while it was considered to be a little fast to be a model, a number of models began to come from the upper classes. In 1924 *Vogue* had reported the current look to be one "of exhausted sophistication".

Marlene Dietrich, who had started her acting career in Germany, moved to Hollywood, and with the help of its make-up artists came to epitomize the sophisticated look, with its flawless porcelain fair skin, red lips and finely drawn eyebrows: a look far removed from the natural look of today. Interestingly enough, although it was an artificial look, it required no more than about six products: foundation, powder, rouge, lipstick, mascara and eyebrow pencil. Very different from the number of products used today to achieve a much more natural look.

Marlene Dietrich was one of the first celebrities to develop a look which, in essence though with variations, she has kept for over forty years. It is an interesting commentary on make-up that some women change their looks with fashion, while others develop a look which they basically keep for most of their lives.

This was the era of the waved hairstyle known as the Marcel wave; it softened the severeness of the Eton crop of the 1920s. It continued to be in fashion right up to the beginning of the Second World War. Pictures of the Duchess of Windsor at the time of her marriage in 1937 show her hair waved on either side of her centre parting.

Max Factor

Max Factor was another cosmetic manufacturer who came to America from Poland at the turn of the century. He had previously worked for the Moscow State Theatre as a make-up artist and he arrived in Hollywood just as silent movies were starting to be made.

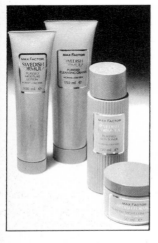

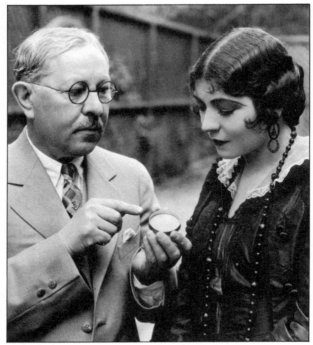

Max Factor was so successful as a stage and screen make-up artist that he was able to sell his products to the public

He made up most of the big movie stars of the day, including Jean Harlow, Mae West and Clara Bow. His most successful products were soon available to the public and he marketed them under the name Society Make-up, in order to give them a classy respectable image. Like most of the cosmetic innovators, he understood the value of endorsement by celebrities, and most of the big stars of the thirties and forties like Bette Davis, Ginger Rogers and Rita Hayworth all promoted Max Factor make-up by unpaid testimonials.

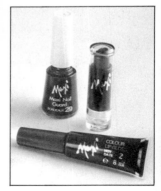

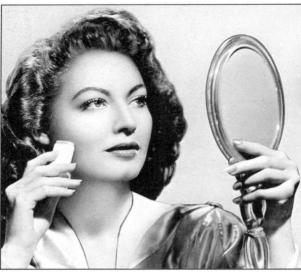

His major contribution to cosmetics was the first grease-paint stick in several flesh tones; this was strong enough to hide skin flaws like freckles, spots and rashes, which showed up badly under the crude studio lights. This product was so popular that he eventually marketed it for the general public and it was in fact the original tinted foundation.

Stars of the era like Ava Gardner, seen here demonstrating the popular Pan-Stik, promoted Max Factor's products by unpaid testimonial

He understood the importance of having an international beauty organization and opened a salon in London in 1936 and later one in Paris.

His son continued the business and was responsible for the introduction of one of the most successful cosmetic products of all time – Pan Cake.

Marlene Dietrich

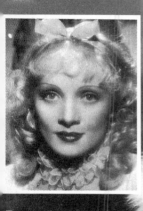

Two styles of Marlene Dietrich: *ingénue* and the look of extreme sophistication which she developed in Hollywood and retained with little variation over many years.

Veronica Lake

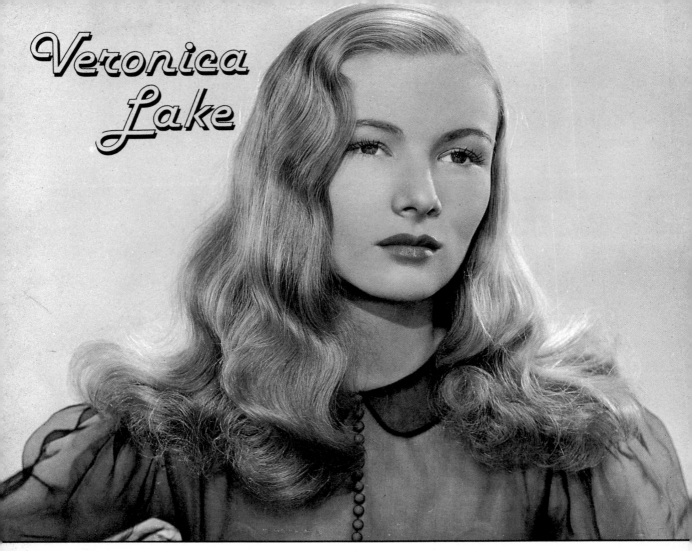

With wartime austerity long hair came back into fashion. Veronica Lake with her peek-a-boo pageboy style caused a certain amount of consternation, because of the number of women who copied her style and had to be persuaded to keep it out of the way while working on munitions. Look at any pictures of the pin-up girls of the war years such as Rita Hayworth, and you can see how long hair returned once more to fashion. Cosmetic manufacturers' research efforts were concentrated on products for the war effort, such as camouflage and skin treatments for burns were given top priority.

As soon as restrictions were lifted, innovations flooded on to the market, and the size of the cosmetic industry has trebled in the last twenty-five years. To conventional products like face cream, tonic, mascara, lipstick and powder, were added first moisturizers, and then a fantastic selection of products to enhance eyes and complexions that could be creamed on, painted on with water, or brushed on dry.

One of the first of these post-war innovations was in the colour range for lipsticks. New petunia-toned pinks burst into fashion: they were the first significant move away from the bright scarlet lips of the twenties and thirties, and started the gradual shift of emphasis towards the eyes.

Charles Revson

Charles Revson entered the cosmetic industry in America in the early thirties, just as it was beginning to enter an era of expansion. He was a born salesman who had tried his hand at a number of different businesses. He felt that there was scope for a really effective nail polish in pretty colours which would replace the only product that was available to put on the nails at that time; this was a paste that was buffed on to nails to give a shine or transparent colour in light, medium and dark shades. It had to be very carefully applied because it usually went streaky.

One of his first innovations was called opaque polish; it went on smoothly and was available in many bright colours. He christened his colours with exotic names like Tropic Sky, Rosy Future, and with a keen sense of timing a delicate pink shade was called Windsor, after the marriage of the Duke and Duchess. It was not long before he spotted what now seems an obvious idea, but which then was truly original: that of matching lipsticks to nail varnishes and vice versa. It was during and after the Second World War that he innovated matching lipsticks and finger tips with names such as Batchelors Carnation, Cherries in the Snow, and Pink Lightning. All these colours were strongly promoted with sexy-looking pictures, such as girls lying on tiger skin rugs.

One of his most famous creations was Blush-On, which he produced in the early sixties. This was a revolutionary concept of rouge: it was a great improvement on the match-to-lipstick pink and crimson cream rouges that

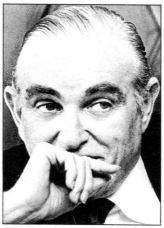

Charles Revson, originator of matching lipstick and nail varnish

warmed up on the skin and looked dolly and unnatural. For Blush-On he used tawny pigments, in easy-to-use powder form, which could be brushed on with a big brush like a man's shaving brush. The use of terracotta colours had first been promoted in Italy, and they gave a subtle glow to the skin. From Blush-On he

Beautiful models promoted Revson's cosmetics

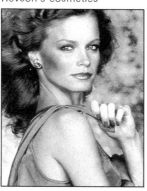

progressed to sticks of tawny colours called Face Gleamers that gave a polished look to the skin.

Just when one or two people in the business felt that some of the newer names in cosmetics might have begun to overtake him, he produced what was probably his most successful creation of all, Charlie. Charlie was not basically breaking new ground in product development, but it was in its concept of the new style of girl he had spotted emerging out of the late sixties. The Charlie girl striding out self-confidently in her well-cut trouser suit represented and appealed to a different buyer: how can one now ever imagine her using one of those heavy boudoir-style scents? No, she was a girl

who wanted original products to conquer new boundaries.

Originally launched as a scent, Charlie was an overnight success; within months it was copied by many of the other beauty houses. And it was not long before Charles Revson, immediately realizing its potential, extended Charlie into a whole range of cosmetics, which in turn have become an outstanding success.

Charles Revson always believed that make-up should be used to enhance one's looks rather than to cover lines and flaws. As he pointed out, a young girl does not wear make-up to make herself look younger, but simply to look good, and that is right for everybody, whatever her age. He believed that creating new products must always be allied to laboratory research; he dismissed "knock-offs" or product copies believing they were never serious competition, because they were always inferior to the original. As he liked to say, "There will always be new ways of doing treatments, new lipstick developments, entirely different looks for make-up."

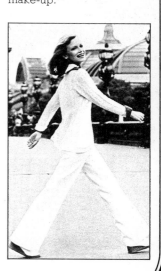

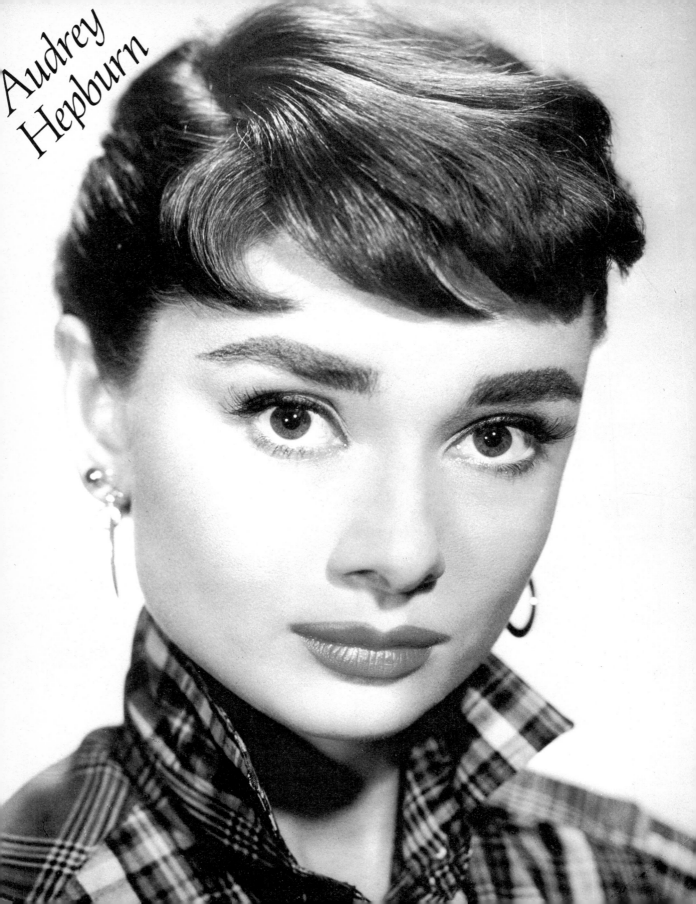

Audrey
Hepburn

By the beginning of the fifties, the eyes had taken over as the focal point of the face. Fluid eyeliner replaced pencilling round the eyes and gave a much stronger emphasis to the shape. Eyebrows returned to their thicker, more natural line after the years of pencil thinness. Young girls whitened out their lips; rouge disappeared. Max Factor's Creme Puff, the first of the combined cream and powder make-ups, came out in 1953 and was an instant success; it became the biggest-selling beauty product ever. It was the first step towards introducing skin tone colours to the fashionable look.

Hollywood's influence began to wane. In its place, European-based cinema stars such as Brigitte Bardot, Sophia Loren and Audrey Hepburn introduced a less stylized glamour. This heralded the beginning of the young developing their own make-up style rather than modelling themselves on their mothers, as they had done previously.

Few films or film stars have had a bigger influence on make-up than Elizabeth Taylor had in *Cleopatra*. This marked the climax of the fashion in which the eye was the most emphasized feature of the face. The extended line at the outer corners of the eye was achieved with black or dark brown liquid eyeliner. Based on the famous head of Nefertiti, the look was an immediate success and quickly taken up by all the leading models of the day. Adapted by Brigitte Bardot and Sophia Loren, the look lived on after its first immediate success. These stars raised the line at the outer corners of the eye, which softened and made the look less stylized. Sophia Loren, like Marlene Dietrich, is another example of a star who has found her style and stuck to it.

The success of the Cleopatra look and of eyeliner also meant the rise of the false eyelash. The strengthening by the use of eyeliner on the top lid and at the sides meant that the eyes would have looked naked without the reinforcement that eyelashes gave them. Suddenly, from being a stage make-up accessory, eyelashes became an everyday beauty product. It was not a coincidence that in Britain the eyelash market was dominated by the Aylott brothers, who for a long time were freelance theatrical and film make-up artists working for companies such as MGM, Warner Brothers and Paramount. False eyelashes had been used for years on the stage, but their introduction to the public came in the wake of the Cleopatra look. Eylure, the Aylott brothers' company, was soon not only marketing eyelashes under its own name, but also manufacturing them for most other cosmetic companies. This continued until the sixties, when the cosmetic manufacturers found that cheaper supplies were available from Vietnam.

False eyelashes were one of the first products introduced to the consumer from the world of stage and film make-up which required too much

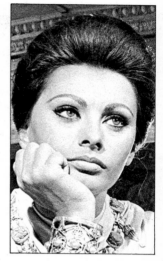

Film stars like Sophia Loren and Brigitte Bardot popularized a more natural glamour than that of their highly stylized Hollywood predecessors.

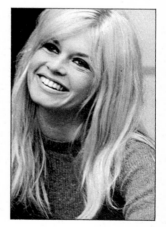

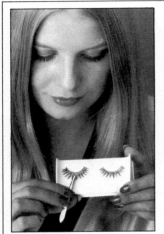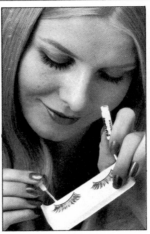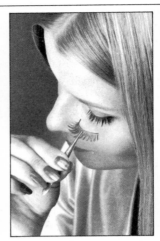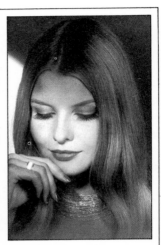

The new definition given to the eyes with the generous use of eyeliner meant a boom in the false eyelash industry.

expertise from the average user. As long as it was fashionable to wear plenty of eyeliner, it was possible to get away with slightly clumsily fitted eyelashes, but as soon as the fashion of eyeliner waned in the sixties, poorly fitted lashes or ones worn too often showed up obviously. Despite these comments, it is remarkable to recall that in one year alone in the late sixties, Eylure sold over five million pairs of eyelashes in Britain.

The late fifties, meanwhile, saw the rise of a rival look: this originated in Italy and was the beginning of the trend towards the more natural look. The credit for evolving this look is usually given to Eve of Roma. It was based on the polished face; no powder, the palest possible lipstick with frosting to give lips added shine, and dark, heavily outlined eyes to give plenty of contrast. A look which was ideal for the growing popularity of sunbathing and Mediterranean holidays, it was quickly picked up by the jet-set at St Tropez, and then popularized by Brigitte Bardot.

The polished face saw the demise of the traditional pink and red rouges which had been matched to lipstick colours. In its place, Eve introduced a liquid terracotta rouge, which she called Roman Glow, and was the forerunner of the tawny toner powder blush-ons introduced by Revlon in the early sixties.

Another important fifties' make-up innovation, taken like so many from the stage, was the use of white powder on the bone above the eyes: its purpose was to increase the distance between the eye and the eyebrow, so

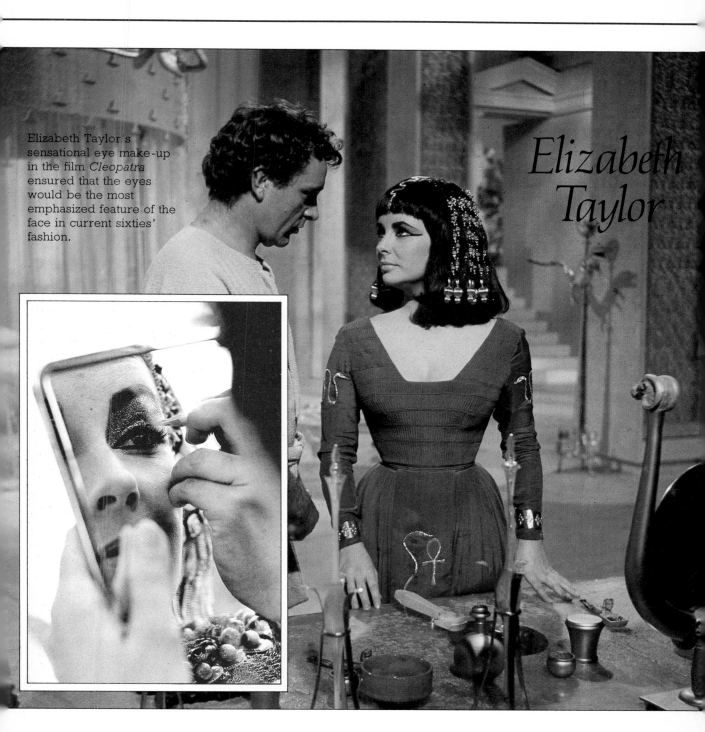

Elizabeth Taylor's sensational eye make-up in the film *Cleopatra* ensured that the eyes would be the most emphasized feature of the face in current sixties' fashion.

Elizabeth Taylor

Eve of Roma

No article on cosmetic innovations would be complete without Eve. She was born in Hungary in the late 1920s, the daughter of cosmetic chemists. She started her career in Rome, when the family fled there in 1946, and she opened a salon in the Via Veneto with her mother and sister.

To Eve, skin care was always as important as make-up: in fact she always said that she envied her elder sister her flawless skin because it enabled her to wear hardly any make-up.

To most people reading this book, Eve is probably the least well known of the innovators and it is difficult for us nearly thirty years afterwards to appreciate today quite how

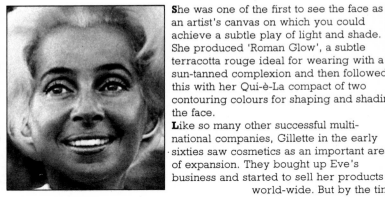

Eve of Roma

She was one of the first to see the face as an artist's canvas on which you could achieve a subtle play of light and shade. She produced 'Roman Glow', a subtle terracotta rouge ideal for wearing with a sun-tanned complexion and then followed this with her Qui-è-La compact of two contouring colours for shaping and shading the face.

Like so many other successful multi-national companies, Gillette in the early sixties saw cosmetics as an important area of expansion. They bought up Eve's business and started to sell her products world-wide. But by the time Eve died in the mid-sixties, it was clear once again that the combination of a multi-national company and cosmetics was not going to work.

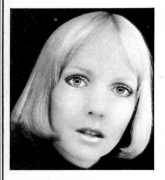

Eve's revolutionary 'polished look'

to Eve who had a thriving salon in Capri in the early fifties. It was here that members of the international set started to adopt her Capri look: shiny skin with large heavily outlined lashed eyes and a pale voluptuous mouth.

It was a look which happened to coincide with a trend away from bright red indelible lipsticks and

it soon became fashionable amongst the young to blot out their lips with panstick make-up.

Eve's was one of the first cosmetic houses to produce clear pale frosted shades in pink, orange or crimson, in what she called a 'Bellissima' combination, which gave the face a completely different focal point, playing up the eyes instead of the mouth.

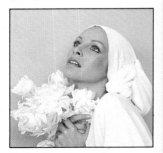

Today the Eve of Roma salon is still in the Via Veneto and carries on the traditions and ideas pioneered by Eve. Like most of the world's leading cosmetic houses, they have a visagiste, Augusta, who creates new make-up looks to complement trends in fashion. The sophisticated bridal make-up pictured above with its light golden foundation and clear, bright lipstick, was created especially by Augusta using Eve of Roma make-up, to go with the current soft, casual look in clothes.

Today's elegant products which may be purchased at Dickins & Jones, London

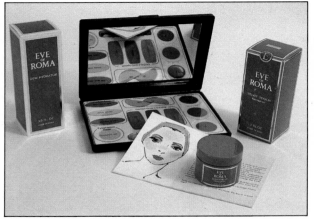

revolutionary the polished look was. In fact it is hard to recall any time in the history of make-up when the objective for the final effect had been anything other than to achieve a pale, whitish matt finish.

Perhaps it wasn't surprising that this new look originated in the Mediterranean where the cult of sunbathing was growing. The credit for turning the sun look into a fashion is generally given

Mary Quant

One of the leading post-war beauty innovators has been Mary Quant. She grew up in the forties and was an art student in the early fifties. She opened her first shop in the King's Road, Chelsea, with clothes that appealed to the young because they were not imitations of the sophisticated styles that were worn by grown-ups. Until Mary Quant, most young girls had always worn versions of what mother wore, and there was no real style for a teenager either in make-up, hair or clothes. Her clothes were mainly in short skinny shapes, and when in the mid-sixties it was suggested that she should give her name to a cosmetic range, she brought many of her fashion ideas into what was a conventional business.

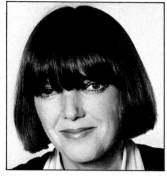

Mary Quant

cosmetic business; she decided it was time for a streamlined range of cosmetics, presented with clear and distinctive packaging and a no-nonsense approach. She realized people were bewildered and bemused by technical terms in the labelling of make-up, so she invented names that described immediately the purpose of the products. In her dictionary, foundation is called Starkers, cleanser Come Clean, tonic Get Fresh, moisturizer Skin Saver, and Cheeky is her name for rouge. Her packaging has the unmistakable Quant hallmark; instead of the conventional gilt with pink or blue trimmings, she has black, white and silver sleek lightweight bottles, streamlined compacts and paintboxes, with her well-known formalized daisy motif. Among her more popular innovations are non-greasy pearlized eye gloss (the modern version of the Vaseline that women used to use to put a shine on their eyelids, in the thirties), tear-proof mascara, and Loads of Lash, used by practically every model in the business for cutting up and putting on in groups of twos and threes between their own lashes.

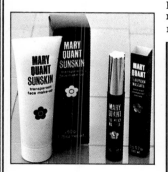

Mary Quant has always said that of all the projects with which she has been associated, she finds cosmetics one of the most stimulating. When she started, she noticed that the models who did her shows used unusual make-up techniques, and that the products which they brought back with them from their trips abroad were mostly superior to those available in Britain. She has been a genuine revolutionary in the

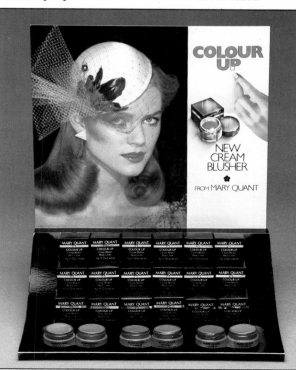

COLOUR UP

NEW CREAM BLUSHER

FROM MARY QUANT

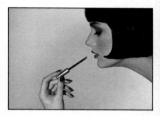

The Quant theory on skin care is also original: she felt all existing products approached the problem from the outside, but as everyone knows, it is what happens inside the body that affects the way your skin behaves. So her Skin Saver cream was sold with Maxi Vitamin pills to boost its effectiveness.

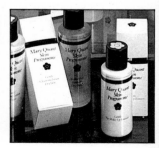

enlarging the look of the eye itself. Every fifties' eyeshadow kit contained a pan of white colour which was meant to be worn with its accompanying blue, green, brown or turquoise shade.

As we move into the sixties, the Italian polished face began to be universally adopted. Eyelashes were still very much in fashion; instead of blatant use of eyeliner, eyeshadow was used to give shape at the outside corner of the eyes, and gave a softer look. Charles Revson introduced Blush-On blushers in soft terracotta colours, so replacing the bright artificiality of rouge; in addition to the powder Blush-On, he introduced a cream stick version in these colours, for achieving the polished look.

Frosting dominated lipstick colours, and was put into nail polishes, foundations and even rouges. Few women understood the significance of frosting. It allowed them to achieve the polished look by counteracting the matt powdery look of make-up. Frosted gleamers on top of foundation gave a beautifully polished look. In fact many women failed to realize that this look was achieved through make-up: they thought it was entirely natural, and felt that they had not spent enough time in the sun to achieve it.

This was a great era for the introduction of new products. Mary Quant was launching her cosmetic range, and was a trendsetter in introducing into her range many products which were based on tricks models used. In many ways she was closer to fashion than many of the large impersonal cosmetic companies. Products like shadower, highlighter, individual lashes cut out from strips and stuck on in ones and twos, were all based on make-up tricks used by leading models. A major Quant innovation, also based on models' habits, was the introduction of brushes for putting on make-up.

By the beginning of the seventies, the natural look had taken over. Products had been developed to remove the obstacles in the way of achieving a natural look: make-up which covered flaws, but still looked transparent; eyeshadows which highlighted the brow-bone, without looking chalky white, in the way that the earlier white shadow powders had; blushers which gave a glow rather than looking rouged on the skin; lipsticks which added colour to the mouth, without looking dry. Paradoxically the natural look meant using more products than ever.

The natural look of today is one of balance between the mouth and the eyes. In this, it is in contrast with the earlier looks of the last sixty years, which had emphasized first the mouth and later the eyes. A major factor in the creation of the natural look has been the advance in the manufacture of much subtler colours. Gone are the harsh pinks and peaches, greens and blues, in favour of beige and gold, freckled brown and subtle pigment colours, which help to achieve natural looking shaping and shading.

Barbara Hulanicki

Like Mary Quant, Barbara Hulanicki was an art student who started as a fashion artist. She then opened a small boutique in the early sixties doing a mail order business in one of the quiet residential streets off Kensington High Street with her husband Stephen FitzSimon. The business boomed and she moved to larger and larger premises. By this time she had established her fashion trade mark which was a revival of art nouveau styles and colours, which she brought up to date and gave her own strong individual style.

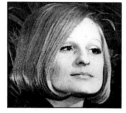

Barbara Hulanicki, the founder of Biba

colours, girls discovered that there were shades which could be used very effectively on the face.

She gave most of her products the simple but stylish presentation which was a feature of all Biba accessories. Her creams and lotions in black pharmacy-style pots and bottles had a sufficiently different image to attract a young user who wanted something quite different from her mother's pink, blue and gilt presented cosmetics.

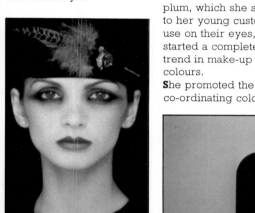

A Biba girl

She introduced the sombre colours of the art deco period for clothes and found that the traditional turquoise, powder-blue, leaf-green eye make-up colours that were available did not go with the monotones such as wine, bottle-green, purple and grey. She therefore introduced a completely new spectrum of cosmetic colours with names such as rust, green bottle, and

plum, which she sold to her young customers for use on their eyes, and this started a completely new trend in make-up colours.

She promoted the idea of co-ordinating colours on the face in the same way as they were co-ordinated in clothes. Cheeks and lips were coloured in wine, plum, and even the murky turquoise she called green bottle. By producing many different tones of these

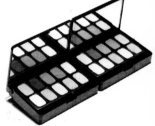

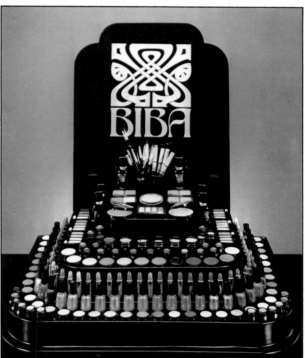

To some extent Barbara Hulanicki was a meteor shooting across the firmament. Now living and working in Brazil, she no longer influences the cosmetic industry in the way she did for that short ten-year span. But for the first time American cosmetic executives reversed the normal trend of bringing fashion colours from America to England, and the Biba colours started a whole new colour trend in the big American make-up companies. Barbara Hulanicki had shown that colours no one had ever previously associated with cosmetics could not only be sold but become overnight sensations. Today's Biba cosmetic range is carried on successfully in Barbara's tradition.

Madeleine Mono

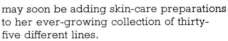

Now that cosmetics have become so much an established part of daily life and are big business, it might well be thought that the development of a new cosmetic range today was beyond the scope of an individual. Many of the leading cosmetic brands are now in the hands of multi-national companies: Max Factor, Helena Rubinstein, Elizabeth Arden and Mary Quant are all owned by major holding companies with many other interests.

All have the financial strength and muscle to surpass a newcomer in advertising and promotion. But cosmetics are not like a lot

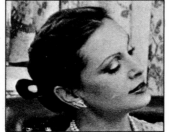

Madeleine Mono loves glitter

of other businesses: it is one which is essentially creative and open to new ideas, the very qualities which large corporations tend not to be good at stimulating.

Characteristically, in the last few years a newcomer has burst upon the scene, and already her cosmetics are among the top sellers in the United States. Madeleine Mono has made her mark in the cosmetic market probably quicker than anyone has done before her.

Now in her mid-forties, Madeleine Mono was born in London. Although her family was firmly established in the rag trade – they own Mono Fashions – she set out to make the stage her career. But then

she married at seventeen and devoted herself to her family, having produced four children in five years. Later her marriage broke up. It was when she married her second husband, Arthur Levene, and went to live with him in New York that, as she says, "my life really began." He suggested that she should start a business, mainly "to give her an interest, and as a hobby". As Madeleine felt that she had always had a natural flair for make-up and women had asked her for years how she achieved that marvellous effect with her eye make-up, she decided that it was an obvious area for her to try.

She started by doing make-up consultations in a friend's salon, and, as she says, "At the end of the first month I was so booked up, and there were a number of products which I used which weren't available in standard ranges, so I thought it was about time I had a go to produce and market Mono ideas."

Having no experience in the cosmetic business she broke all the so-called rules and started with just one make-up product. It was a mini-stick of black Kajal to put on the inside of the eye. She called it Indian Eyes, and took it to the big New York stores herself. Bloomingdales sold it very successfully, and were soon re-ordering.

Only she and Barbara Hulanicki have achieved their initial success entirely with make-up. Possibly this is because they are the two most recent innovators and their success reflects the important role that make-up now plays. My guess is that Madeleine

may soon be adding skin-care preparations to her ever-growing collection of thirty-five different lines.

Madeleine's most successful line at the moment is what she calls "Twinkling Glimmering Shimmering Blinking Body Glitter". She describes it as a "delicate gel, marvellously fragranced with rose-petal oil, and laced with thousands of minute shimmering particles that glisten and gleam all over the skin. Body Glitter is celestial glamour; a universe of night-time drama."

Customers are recommended to wear Body Glitter to a disco, and in fact it is the coincidence of designing a product which is exactly right for the current disco boom and the vogue for glittering clothes in shiny fabrics that has made this product into a sell-out success. Body Glitter should be spread sparingly on to your skin – face, shoulders, arms or legs.

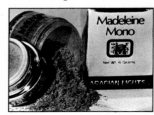

I asked Madeleine what were the main ingredients of the Mono face for the eighties, and according to her American make-up artist Jim Kennedy it will be a gleaming face, the eyes highlighted with iridescent powder, yet still defined with plenty of Indian Eyes Kajal, and on the lids Arabian Lights shadows – "gold drenched powder colours that radiate beauty and warmth".

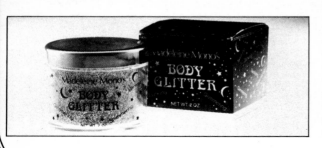

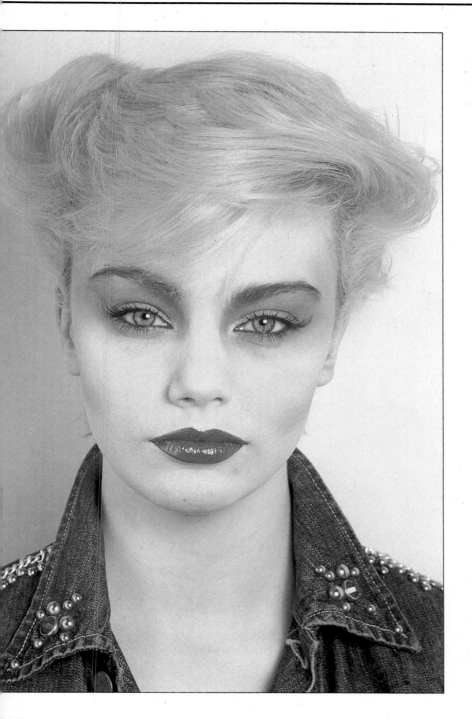

80s?

It is not easy to predict the look of the eighties, nor indeed to predict make-up trends for any new decade. It is never a logical progression of the current look. So many factors determine the course of fashion: although beauty has become a £150 million a year business in Britain alone, and many of the largest industrial companies such as ICI and Unilever are all involved in it, the inspiration for the new look will almost certainly come from an individual.

Accordingly, I spoke to several young freelance artists who do make-ups for photography in magazines and newspapers. Most of them had been inspired by the exotic effects achieved by the punk rockers, with whitened complexion and startling colours on eyes and lips. I asked one of them, Alistair, to do a make-up which had the eighties look.

He started with a bleached-out skin tone using theatrical white foundation and powder by Max Factor. For the eyes he blended Ultima II shadow colours Spun Gold Bronze and Spun Silver Pink with Orange and Rose eye-shadows by Cosmetics à la Carte. The lipstick is a mixture of Nos 37 and 83, also by Cosmetics à la Carte.

BEST IMAGES

Some of us are born more beautiful than others. But there are far fewer of us born that way than you might think, and having worked for over thirty years with many of the top models, I can assure you that nine times out of ten the most attractive women you see owe as much to self-awareness, self-discipline, personality and knowledge, as they do to natural attributes.

Nothing is more instructive than looking at pictures of well-known film stars and models taken before and after thay have become famous. Marlene Dietrich, Marilyn Monroe and Jean Shrimpton all bear out this point. Of course it is true that these girls have had the advantage of having the full weight of the studio make-up and hair experts behind them, but the rest of us can still do a lot to make the best of our looks.

I know many women who look at top models and say, "I wish I could look like that." Seldom do they realize the time and trouble that the model has taken in working out her best and worst points and emphasizing or camouflaging them. Nearly all of us have at least one friend who makes up well, and you can be sure she has spent time thinking about it and experimenting with various looks. Magazines, particularly some of the popular weekly ones, give a very comprehensive beauty service, and you can pick up a lot of ideas and tips from their beauty articles. But there is no real substitute for being shown by an expert; unfortunately standards vary considerably and there are few good make-up experts out of London.

There is one useful tip I can give: Selfridges hold their Beauty Playground for two weeks every year after Christmas. The idea is to have an area in the store removed from the cosmetic counter where you can try on any product you wish: in this area of the store there is no selling. In fact it is impossible to buy a product here even if you wish to; to buy you have to walk down to

Lyndall Hobbs is the lady responsible for the revival of this fifties' favourite – petunia pink lipstick, which Cosmetics à la Carte made up specially for her about two years ago. This particular shade of petunia lipstick is No. 69, and Lyndall puts it on with a brush. She emphasizes her eyes with brown powder shadow, applies a touch of translucent pressed powder, no foundation and Cosmetics à la Carte orchid blusher to tone with the lipstick.

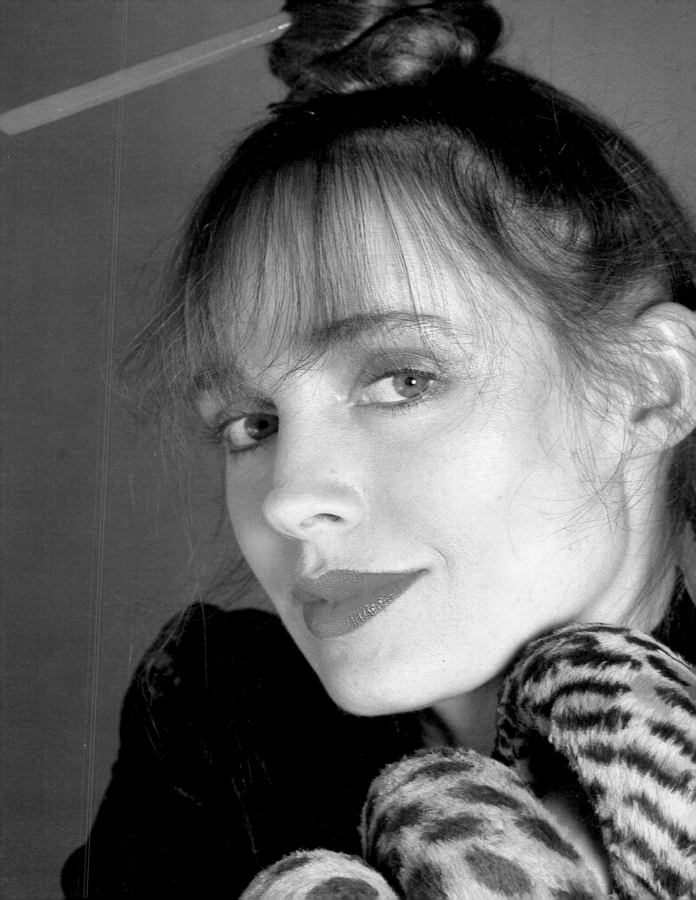

the cosmetic department. This means you cannot be pressurized into buying while you are in the Playground.

Each year since it started four years ago, Selfridges have asked me to take part with three of my girls – to give independent advice about the cosmetics of the twenty or so manufacturers who attend with their own make-up artists. I have found when I have been in the Playground that a lot of the women who come there are middle-aged and feel that they need to do something about their looks. Somehow the informal atmosphere of the Playground, the absence of the hard-sell, the knowledge that there is no way anyone is going to know whether you buy or not, all gives confidence to anyone who is a little unsure of herself. My observation is that the Playground has been a success; in particular it seems to bring into touch with up-to-date make-up ideas many women who have let them slip by. It really does offer a unique opportunity to experiment and try on make-up. Now that it has become established, perhaps it will be adopted by stores out of London. I certainly believe there is a need for it.

Realizing your full potential is to a much greater extent than people suspect largely a question of determination. I can think of no better example of someone who has done her best to improve her looks than Maria Callas. If you see any picture of her right up to her mid-twenties, you will see a rather plump Greek girl, and I am sure that most of us, had we looked like her, would not have made the effort required to overcome the problem; instead, we would have sunk back into the consolation of eating sticky cakes and general over-indulgence in food. But the very fact of her success as a singer and her professional desire to be one of the great opera stars, together with an awareness which was ahead of her time, that acting and therefore appearance would be critical in reaching a new pinnacle of success in the opera, drove her to achieve what many women consider to be almost a miracle. Look at the pictures of her after thirty, and you will see an attractive, sophisticated, successful woman who seemed as if she had been born with so many advantages over other singers.

It is easier to achieve such a transformation if you have the motivation of success in a career and a very clear ultimate goal; of course, it is much tougher to motivate yourself when the biggest event in your day is a visit to the supermarket or collecting your children from school. Apathy is a hurdle that many women have to overcome if they want to make the best of themselves.

Many women suffer from needless inhibitions when it comes to improving their appearance with the use of make-up. In this respect my clients fall into two main categories. There are those who have been brought up in families

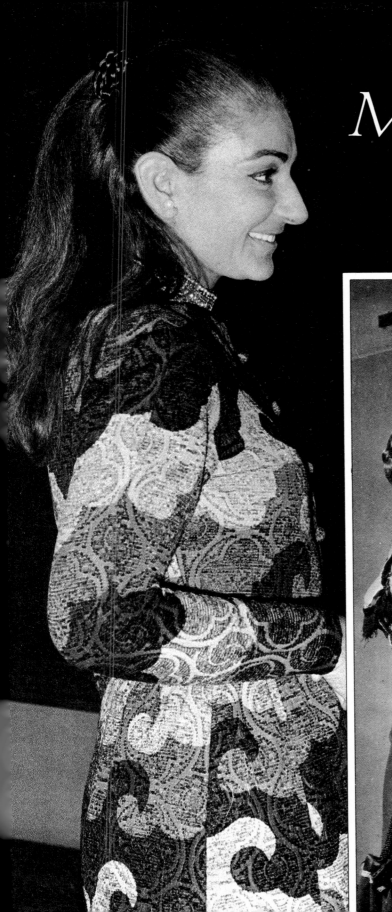

Maria Callas

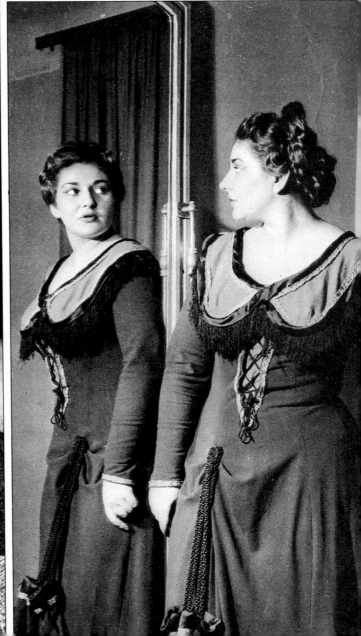

where make-up is regarded as quite acceptable, and others whose families have frowned on its use. Often when these women try using make-up for the first time, their faces feel uncomfortable, and they become shy and self-conscious about how other people look at them. If they persevere, they will find that they gain confidence from looking their best.

Similarly, I have often spoken to Bernice Weston, who started Weight Watchers in this country, and who in making it such a successful venture has done so much to show overweight people that it is possible not only to slim, but also to remain slim. Bernice always says that women who, when they were fat, took no interest in make-up and clothes because they felt it was a world which was closed to them, took an immediate interest in themselves once they had begun to lose weight.

I have judged several Weight Watchers competitions for Bernice in the past, and like everyone else I am always fascinated by seeing men and women who have lost eight or ten stone. Yes, I have seen women who weighed over twenty stone, and have slimmed themselves down to under twelve. Talking to them, I have always been surprised at their sudden interest in make-up and what it can do for them.

Make-up really does help us to make the most of our good points, hide many of our less good points, and in fact helps us look and feel our best. As in any branch of fashion, looks come and go; make-up helps us adapt our faces to the fashion. Using make-up does not mean that you have to look "made-up", wearing heavy "Cleopatra" eyes and red lipstick. Part of the art of making up is to know what it is that makes you look made-up: for instance, false eyelashes, which are currently very much out of fashion, black and dark brown lines with pale blue or green shadow on eyes, floury pinky white face, and pale frosted pink lips are all points which give you away. It does mean that you can give yourself high cheekbones, dark eye-lashes, and an even complexion. In fact many of the most natural faces around today owe much of their success to face shapers, shaders, cheek highlighters, blushers, eye glosses, eye crayons, eye tints, kohl pencils, lip tints and glosses – and yet they still look natural.

As I have said before, beauty is so much an attitude of mind, the more attractive you look the more attractive you want to look; the less attractive you feel the less interested you become and gradually the world of beauty and make-up becomes closed to you. All the women photographed on these pages by Pat Booth have taken time and trouble to make themselves look good. They all have strong views about beauty which are often very different. But what they have in common is that it is a subject which interests them and one to which they have given considerable thought.

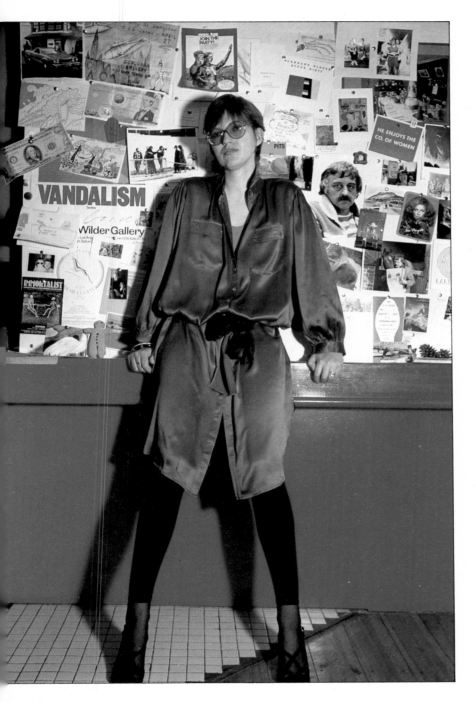

Almost as important a part of looking good is feeling good, and that is why – if you have managed to master the art of how to put on make-up – you will find that you feel more confident and almost certainly more attractive.

Janet Street Porter, TV personality and former writer on the *Evening Standard*, is a classic example of how to make the best of yourself. I am sure Janet would be the first to admit that she was not born beautiful. A very tall girl, she has mastered most of the tricks of looking good. In particular she has had the courage and personality to develop a style of her own.

To start with, she has a dramatic and stylish haircut: it is impossible to stress enough the importance of having your hair well cut. This is almost always the right starting off point.

She is also a shining example to any girl who feels that she was born unlucky because she has to wear glasses. Like Janet you you can turn your glasses into much more than a fashion accessory. With these becoming big frames, which can be an expression of your personality, you could well copy Janet – she has several pairs in different colours and wears them according to her mood.

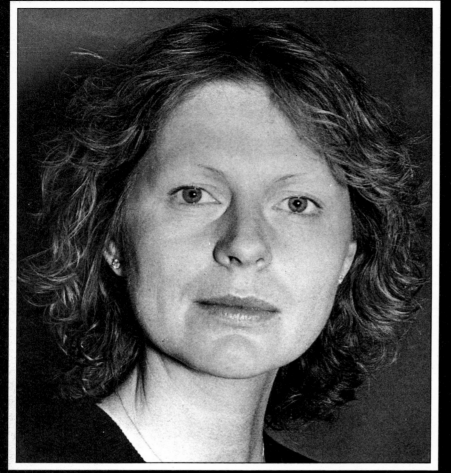

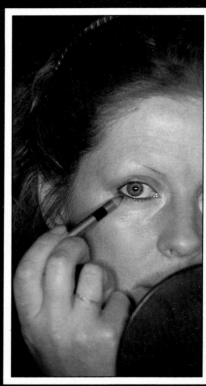

· ·· before

Paulene Stone

Paulene Stone, who for years was a top model and was married to Laurence Harvey, is one of the most attractive women you are likely to meet today. She knows her good and less good points and how make-up helps to deal with them. Her success in getting the very best out of her looks can be seen by contrasting the picture of her with no make-up with that showing her as she normally appears wearing make-up.

Paulene believes that blusher is her most important beauty accessory. "I think I look absolutely hideous without it, in fact my friends always ask me if I am feeling ill. Blusher gives me

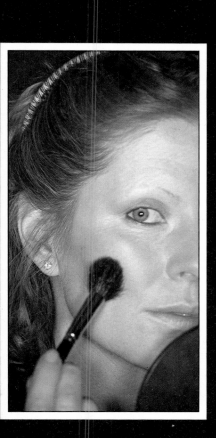

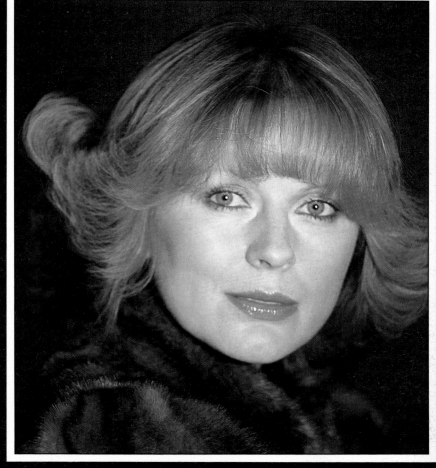

after ...

Jill Bennett

Actress Jill Bennett has an unusually distinctive face, but it is not what you would describe as classically beautiful. As you can see from her picture, she knows how to make herself look outstandingly attractive. She believes the right foundation is what matters most to her and has discovered that one of the secrets of a natural-looking make-up is to go for a beige colour which will give a golden tone to the skin. She relies on having her blond hair highlighted very finely to keep the fairness which is so much part of her image, and has her hair done regularly by Wendy at Shades in Thurloe Place in Kensington.

For our photograph Jill is wearing a golden beige foundation, Elizabeth Arden's Toasty Beige Flawless Finish, with Revlon's Frosty Sienna blusher and Innoxa's Truly Peach to highlight the top of her cheekbones, underneath the outer corner of the eyes. Eyeshadow colours are achieved with Lancôme's Pewter Pencil and Elizabeth Arden's Golden Grape and Charles of the Ritz's Smokey Blue shadows. Her lipstick is Elizabeth Arden's Bronze Lamé.

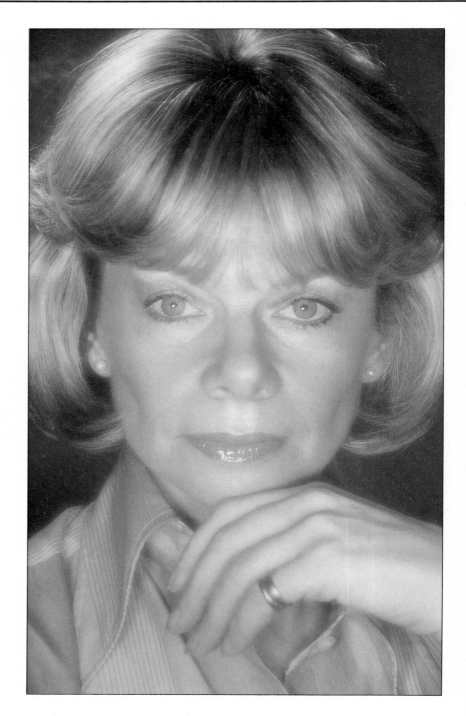

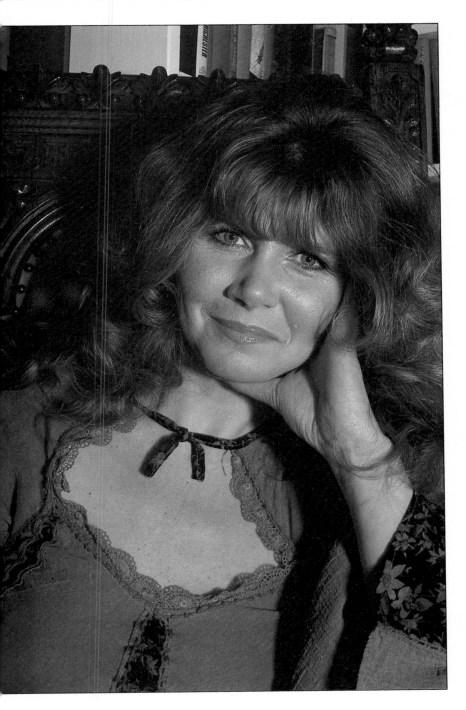

Jilly Cooper

Jilly Cooper would not claim to be conventionally beautiful, and in fact has probably spent less time thinking about her looks than the other personalities photographed in these pages. With a strong personality, she relies on this as much as on her looks.

Jilly warned make-up girl Sarah that she could not bear having her face made up because she found the more she put on, the worse it looked. She had only four or five make-up items which she reckoned was quite sufficient. However, Sarah used a total of eleven products and Jilly found that her make-up looked surprisingly more natural than she had expected.

Sarah used Charles of the Ritz's foundation Sirtaki, with Face Place Powder and Brown Shader and Mary Quant's Toffee Blushbaby. Her eye make-up included Guerlain's Champagne Cream Shadow with Fabergé's Babe Roast Chestnut and Sugar and Spice, Max Factor's Brownish Black mascara and Galitzine's Brown kohl pencil, and Mary Quant's Peach Ultra Lights on the brow-bone. The lipstick is Mary Quant's Chilli Crush.

Bianca Jagger

Bianca Jagger is one of the most photographed celebrities today. Born in Nicaragua, her face has all the dramatic beauty of South America and she is unquestionably one of the great stylists.

For this picture her make-up was done by Barbara Daly, one of the leading make-up artists in this country. She was one of the first to use artists' crayons to widen the limited scope of make-up colours available in the early 1960s. This has led to the profusion of eye-colour crayons available today.

For Bianca's make-up Barbara used Clinique's Almond Beige Balanced Make-up Base, and Boots No.7 Peach Bloom Peach Soft Blush. On the eyes she blended Boots No.7 Shadowmists Brownie and Blackbird, and used Clinique's Glossy Black Glossy brush-on mascara. The lipstick is Clinique's Golden Plum Different lipstick, with their Black Honey Lip Gloss over the top. As Barbara says, "I think Bianca has so much personality she can afford to underplay her make-up".

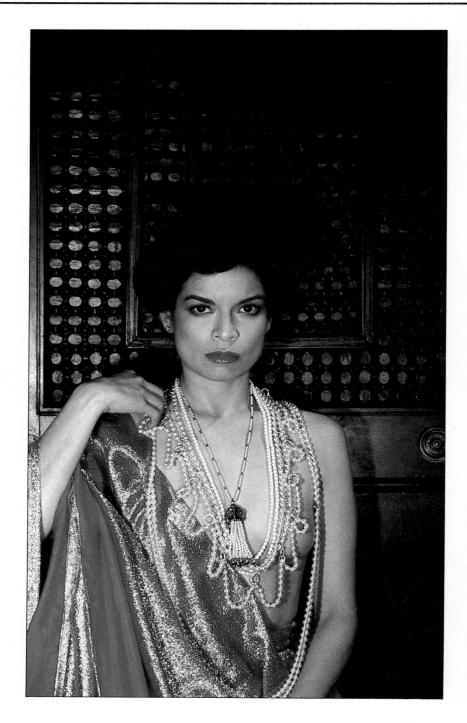

Zandra Rhodes

Another very forceful personality, and one whose looks are in no way conventional, is Zandra Rhodes, the well-known designer. She has her own highly individual ideas on make-up and she has no inhibitions about the amount of make-up she wears. The products she uses are meant to show. With her innate artistic skill she applies bright petunia pink blusher to give a fabulous dramatic effect, and takes a black make-up crayon to draw in a zig-zag contour line around the outside of her face, which outlines the way her hair frames it.

About her hair Zandra says, "I change colour frequently, using those bright vegetable dyes. It gives you plenty of scope for using colours in your make-up, and I think that you don't want to take it all too seriously – nowadays people expect me to look the way I do."

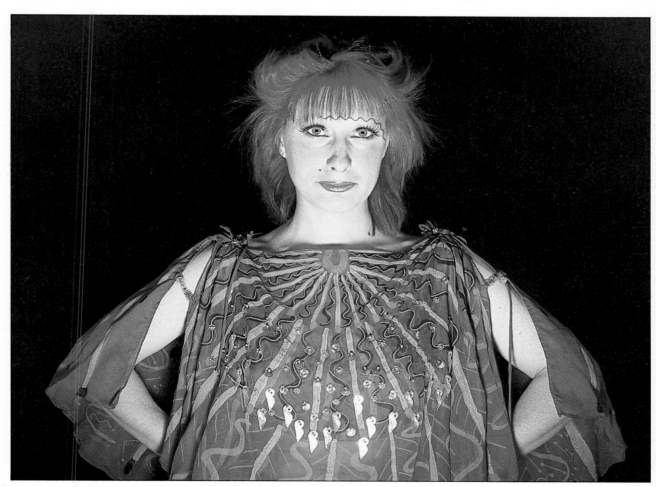

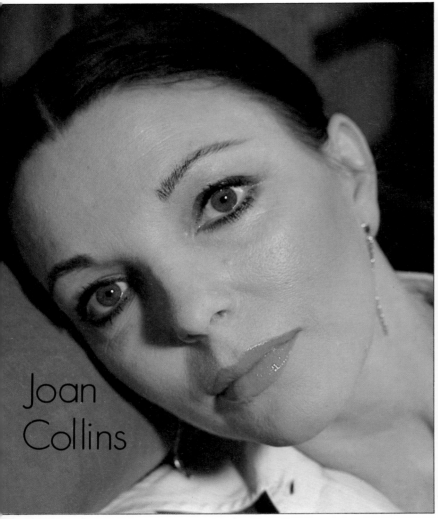

Joan Collins

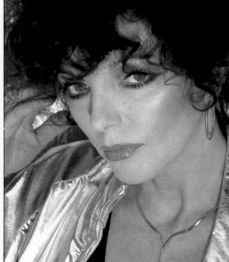

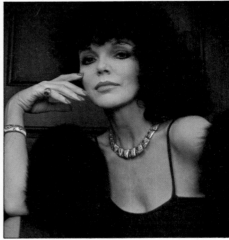

All the personalities we have photographed and discussed so far have developed definite personalities and looks of their own. But if you can master the art of make-up, you can give yourself considerable choice about the type of image you wish to project.

We asked two well-known actresses, Joan Collins and Susan George, to let us work with them in producing three different looks. These pictures should give you a good idea of the scope open to you.

No one is more aware of what can be achieved with make-up than Joan Collins. In the larger picture she emphasizes the classical regularity of her features by adopting a sleek hairstyle. (*Top right*) For a sophisticated mood Joan uses make-up to give added definition to her eyes.

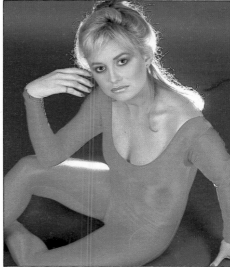

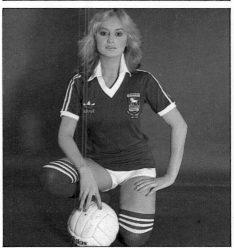

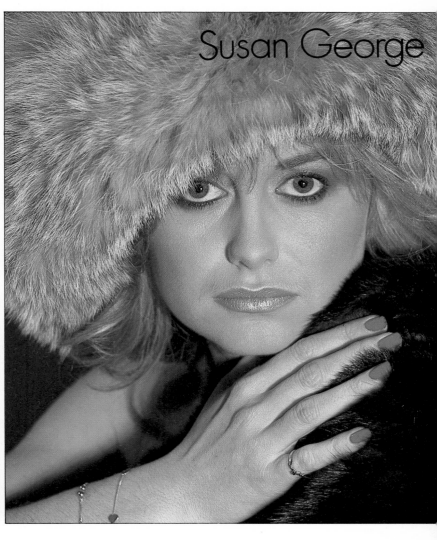

Susan George

(Below left) For a striking evening look, she skilfully highlights and shades her dramatic cheekbones to counteract the flattening effect of artificial lighting.

(Above) Susan George shows how effectively you can adapt your looks to suit the clothes you are wearing. In the larger picture we see her looking sophisticated in a large fur hat. As an actress she knows how to emphasize her looks using a darker foundation and plenty of face shader and blusher. (Top and bottom left) In more relaxed and informal moods, Susan wears a red cat suit and is dressed for the sporting life. For these two pictures her make-ups were soft and more natural looking.

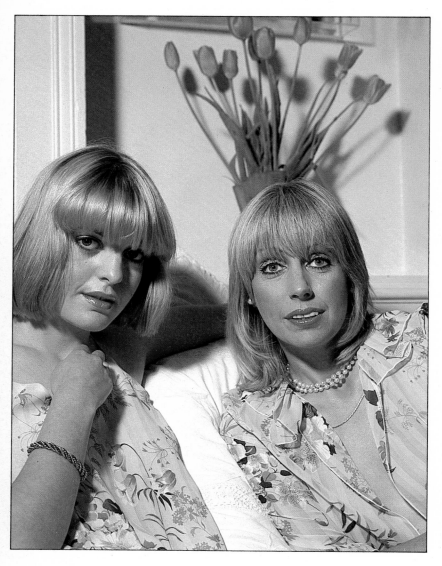

One of the most dramatic changes in make-up today is that our faces no longer necessarily proclaim our age. In fact I know many mothers and daughters who look far more like sisters.

Suki Marlow and her nineteen-year-old daughter Laura (*above*) have a strong link in the way they wear their hair. They both go to the same hairdresser, Mary at Crispin in Kensington. For Pat Booth's picture they were made up by Sarah at the Face Place:

"I used the currently fashionable aubergine, plum and pink eyeshadow colours on both of them: these tones are quite hard to wear unless you have big eyes, and in both cases the colours looked very effective."

Like many mothers and daughters today, actress Nanette Newman and her twenty-year-old daughter, Sarah Forbes (*opposite*), share a lot of beauty ideas. Both are original in their use of make-up: while their "musts" include blusher, mascara and lip gloss, neither uses face powder, eyeshadow or lipstick.

Their make-ups for the photograph were by Sarah of the Face Place. On Nanette she used Lancôme No. 3 Maquimat foundation, Revlon Frosty Rose Blush On, Charles of the Ritz Softshine and Seagreen Mist Eye Shadow Pommades, Orlane Black eye crayon and Babe Terracotta, a coloured lip gloss. Sarah has on Germaine Monteil's Ivory Beige Superglow foundation, Face Place Shadower, Quant Toffee Blusher, Coty Bisque Highlighter, Charles of the Ritz Softshine and Khaki eyeshadow pommades, Miss Selfridge No.1 Gold and Princess Galitzine's Silvery Green eye crayon. The lipstick is Mary Quant's Chilli Crush.

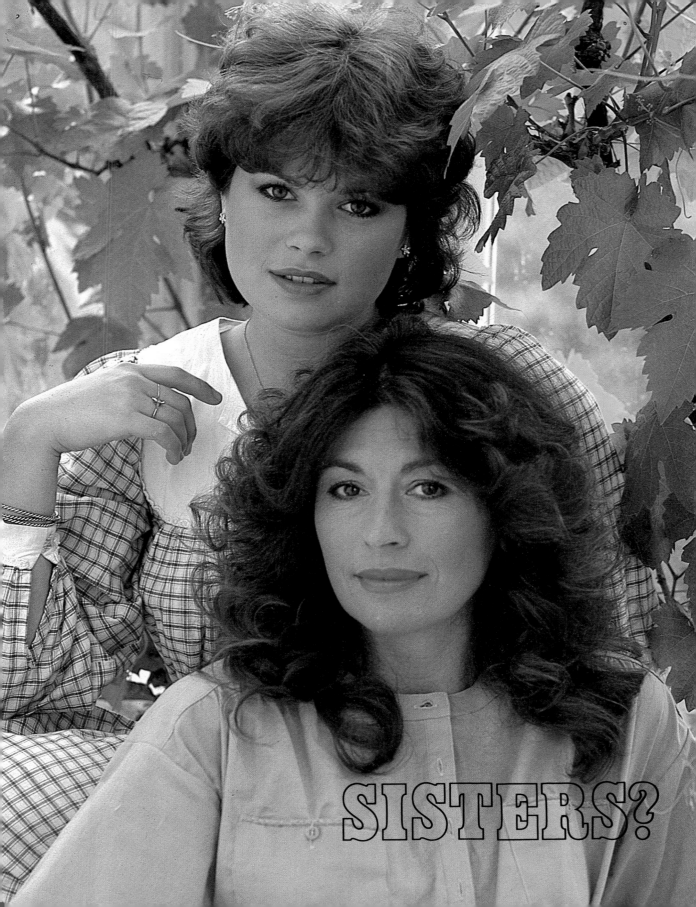

SISTERS?

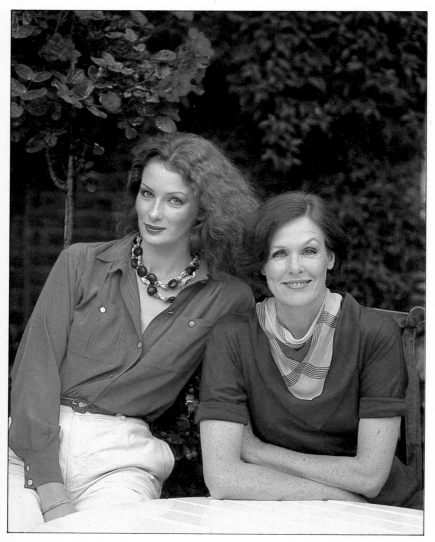

mix to get the effect I want.''

Her daughter Wendy, who is a successful model in New York, has inherited her mother's good looks. She has naturally curly hair which she wears long on to her shoulders. She shampoos it every few days using a natural herb shampoo by Leonard and his special herb conditioner.

Both mother and daughter use Ponds Cold Cream: they find it acts as an effective cleanser and does not irritate their skin. Wendy is also a fan of a moisturizing product called Creme Simon. Of course, Jenny has one great advantage which, if you are not born with it, is difficult to achieve: she has marvellous natural facial bone structure.

Another striking example chosen and photographed by Pat Booth are actress Vivienne Ventura and her teenage daughter (*opposite*). Both capitalize on their natural good looks by using the minimum of make-up, which is the big advantage of being born a brunette. They both play up their eyes with subtle shadows to give soft emphasis and use delicate pink on their lips with plenty of gloss. They use warm golden complexion tones which flatter their fair skins and act as a striking contrast to their dark hair.

A much admired mother, with a grown-up daughter, Jennifer Hocking is former *Harpers & Queen* magazine fashion editor. Jenny has a very simple philosophy for not looking her age. ''Keep your make-up simple and see that you wear your hair in a style that you can manage yourself.'' She cuts and colours her own hair and wears very little foundation, but believes in using make-up to enhance her eyes. ''I have lots of shadows in different colours which I blend and

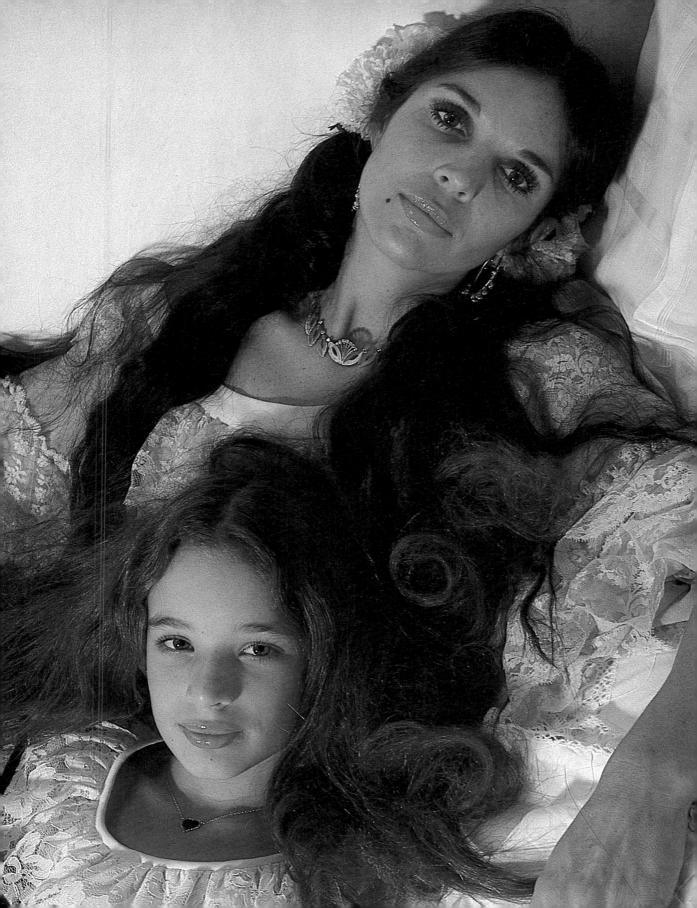

I find that one of the most intriguing aspects of beauty is that women who look good fall into two categories. The first are those who change their style with fashion. If straight hair is fashionable, they will adopt it, and then when curly hair supersedes it, they will in turn go curly; at the same time they change their make-up. The second are women who having found a certain look retain it. You might think that this would date them, and according to many rules it should. There are many examples, however, of women who have so developed their style and manage to carry it off so well, that in no way do they look dated. I believe that this is an intuitive approach and the pictures opposite say more than words.

As a generalization you will find that most top models who stay at the top adjust their looks to the changing fashions. They have to, because fashion photography is about fashion. If you look at pictures of top models you will find that over a period they vary their hair and faces considerably. Petula Clark is an example from show business who has kept her looks very much in tune with fashion. In fact there are few show business personalities who have been at the top for as long as Petula Clark, yet no one gets tired of her face

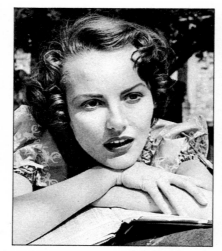

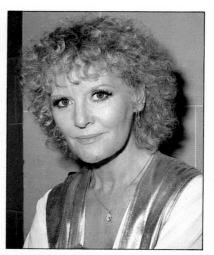

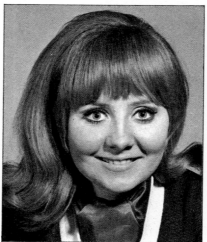

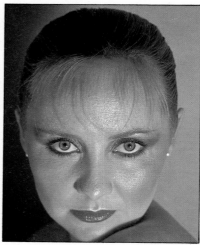

because she has managed to adapt her style to keep looking permanently fresh and contemporary. Here we see two examples, one from her unsophisticated teenage days and, right, her current look of a relaxed, confident star.

Pop star Lulu is another good example of a successful change of style. She became a star at fifteen in the film *To Sir With Love* when she sang the hit song "*Shout*". In those days she was known for her "girl-next-door" looks, flicked-up hairstyle and a dash of pale lipstick. She is now married to top hairdresser John Freida who has encouraged her to develop a more sophisticated style.

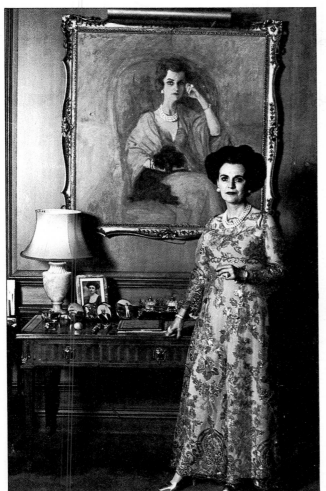

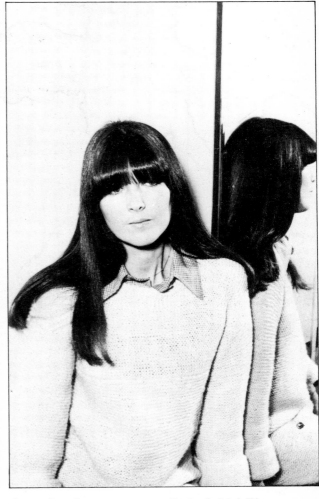

A leading non-style-changer is Margaret, Duchess of Argyll. A top deb when she came out in the thirties, she has always retained her own style. She says that you can only do this successfully if you know yourself well. "I have kept the same style but with modifications: obviously it depends on a number of factors such as your silhouette, the colouring of your hair and keeping your legs in shape. Yes, I think I am recognizable by the way I wear my hair and I hardly ever wear hats".

Kathie McGowan, the star of the sixties T.V. show *Ready Steady Go,* hasn't altered her style or her hair since she was fourteen. Now in her early thirties, she still wears it straight falling on to her shoulders with a fringe. Keeping the same hairstyle imposes a special discipline on her figure: "I realize that it is important that the rest of me looks right and so I take good care to keep my weight down. I'm still size ten in clothes: whenever I need to I go on a diet."

Visagistes

As an ultimately inspiring example of looks that can be achieved through a mastery of the art of make-up we are including a reference to the work of the visagistes.

The visagistes are professional make-up artists who work for the major cosmetic houses, and because they make up models for photographic sessions for magazines and newspapers, they are to a large extent the arbiters of looks in the cosmetic world.

One of the first beauty houses to employ a visagiste was Elizabeth Arden. Pablo was trained in Elizabeth Arden's salon in Paris, and in the 1950s he revolution- ized the use of colour. In fact, one of the main functions of the visagiste has been to update the colours produced by the cosmetic company they work for. A good visagiste should create a new palette of shades every season to complement the current fashion colours.

It was the influence of the visagistes that inspired the introduction of colour- coordinated eyeshadows. Early eyeshadow kits

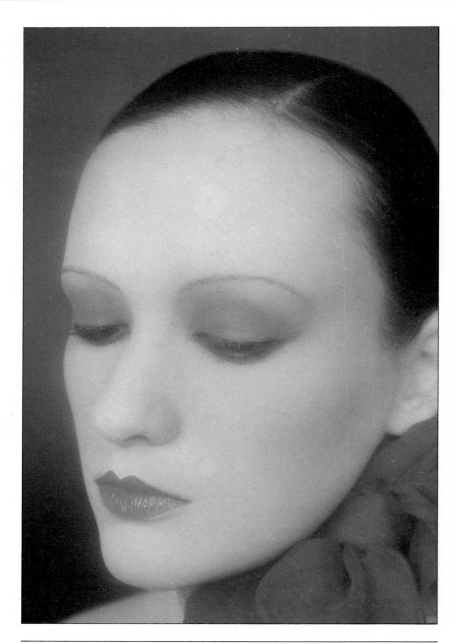

Two contrasting looks on one of Serge's favourite models, Isabelle Weingarten; one a classic look and the other a more dramatic interpre- tation of make-up inspired by a French painter, Fernand Léger.

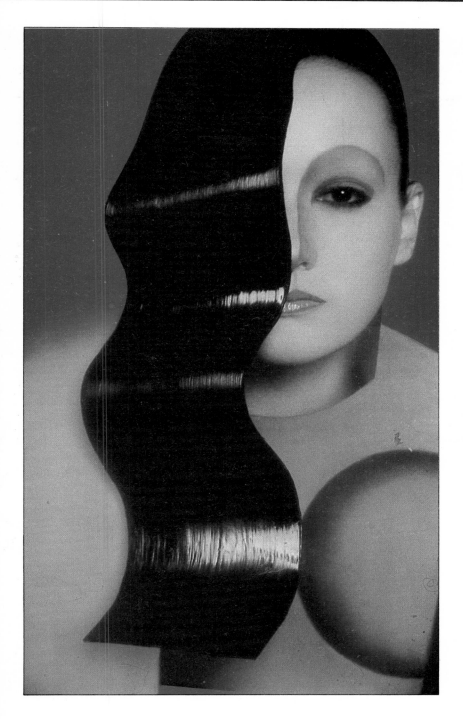

contained four unrelated tones which were meant to be worn separately. The visagistes realized that a more dramatic eye make-up could be produced if the colours were coordinated so that they could be worn together.

Max Factor have had several well-known visagistes, the most famous of whom was a Belgian called Gil, who created make-ups for most of the top international houses. Douglas Young is another well-known Max Factor make-up artist who has been with the company for many years, and was in fact their theatrical director in London. He has been responsible for many of their most successful colours.

One of the most original visagistes is Serge Lutens of Christian Dior. A Frenchman who started as a hairdresser, he began working in the early 1960s with a number of top Paris photographers who persuaded him to do the make-up as well as the hair. Serge has worked for most of the top glossy magazines, and he is probably the most startlingly original of all the visagistes. He makes dramatic use of an assortment of mediums as part of his make-up. He sticks broken coloured glass, dead flies, and sand on to his models, but the effect is always fascinating.

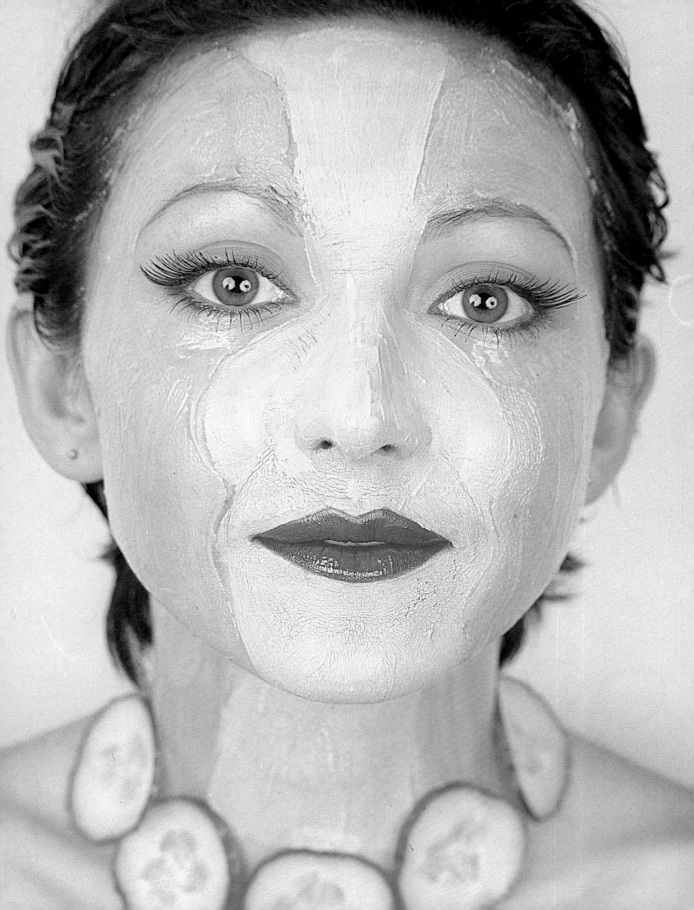

SKIN CARE

Your face is one of your most valuable possessions and like many other possessions you have, it needs looking after. It is my observation that the women who spend the most time and trouble looking after their faces tend to have smoother, less lined complexions. It is something I often tell women who ask me if I think it is important to use skin-care preparations.

Make-up is not the only type of beauty aid which has been used since the beginning of civilization. Herbs, which are enjoying a revival in terms of their use in beauty, have been used since the beginning of time for both medicinal and beauty purposes. Increasingly we are discovering all over again what our ancestors knew so well – that there are special beneficial properties inherent in so many herbs, especially for improving the skin. Natural ingredients are also in vogue, having been used throughout history. For instance, women in Ancient Rome used eggs for face packs; these were later used by the women of the court of Versailles, and were of course the basis of many Victorian recipes for skin care. The Ancient Egyptians were great users of mud packs for the face, the mud coming from the rich soil of the Nile, and to all intents and purposes the treatment they gave themselves was very much the same as the mud face pack you can have in any salon today.

Let me say straight away that neither science nor nature has yet produced a miracle cream which will give a woman of fifty the same unwrinkled skin as her teenage daughter. But that is not an argument for doing nothing and I firmly believe that there is a lot you can do to withstand the worst evidence of ageing in your skin.

Often I meet people who say that they cannot understand why we do not allow our skin to look after itself. Many women have strange ideas about their skin, such as leaving off make-up for a day in order to give it a rest, and not putting face cream on at night in order to let their skin breathe. Of course it is true that the skin is designed to be able to keep itself in good order naturally, but the ravages caused by sun and harsh weather, quite apart from man-made irritants of modern life such as pollution and the drying effects of central heating and air conditioning, can interfere with the natural functioning of the skin. Unfortunately it is only when things go wrong, such as dryness, chapping, too much oil with blackheads and spots, that we become aware of the need to look after our skin. The ultimate reason for looking after our skin is that most of us wish to delay signs of ageing.

One of the main obstacles to skin care is that when you are young you are seldom aware of the problems ahead, and find it hard to believe that your skin will change as much as it does. For instance, few people realize the extent to which dehydration of our skin takes place as we get older, but it is frequently not until a woman reaches the mid-thirties that the little lines that we associate with ageing become noticeable. Unfortunately modern living habits are doing nothing to help. Three of the chief enemies of an unwrinkled skin are air conditioning, central heating and the sun; in fact, the very same things which spoil your furniture. Air conditioning is even more damaging to the skin than central heating. Both are dehydrating to the skin, air conditioning very much so. If you work in an air-conditioned office, I would state quite categorically that you must do something to look after your skin. If you do nothing, you may not notice much effect as long as you are under thirty, but once over forty I can assure you that you will find your skin dry and more wrinkled than that of your contemporaries. The sun, too, both burns and dries our northern skins and with our current cult for sunbathing, it is necessary to take steps to prevent its worst effects.

Women are always asking me what difference science has made to skin care. This is not an easy question to answer. Science has affected skin care in two main areas. First, machinery: some of the new developments in machinery for facials have certainly meant that more effective facials can be given to older skins. The second area, which seems to concern women most, is that of skin creams. These basically originate from traditional herbal recipes, and as I mentioned in chapter 2, many were introduced by beauty therapists from Central Europe.

Originally the main role of the chemist in cosmetic formulation was to give a better consistency and more stability to herbal recipes. But in the last forty years, as more and more scientists have become involved in the industry, they have widened their role to see if they can solve some of the problems posed by nature in the ageing process.

Some people are very strongly opposed to the chemist's or scientist's influence in formulating creams. These views are frequently held by people who are dedicated herbalists and feel that any interference with nature must be detrimental. Herbalists believe that no cures can take effect immediately, that the body must be assisted to help itself and that nature's remedies need time. They tend to resent the scientist's attempt to quicken up the effect of a product and disagree with the idea of a scientist formulating a different product for each type of skin. In fact most cosmetic manufacturers seem to me to combine the best of each approach. My reservations about the herbalist's view is that products formulated without any scientific additions do tend to have a somewhat crude consistency and a short life.

It is certainly true to say that night creams are beneficial when you reach your early forties. They give added moisture to a dry skin; but more important, scientists have utilized their technology to incorporate ingredients that have a noticeable skin-plumping effect, and so soften the appearance of wrinkles.

In order to care for your skin you need to understand its structure: this diagram is a simplified cross section of the skin.

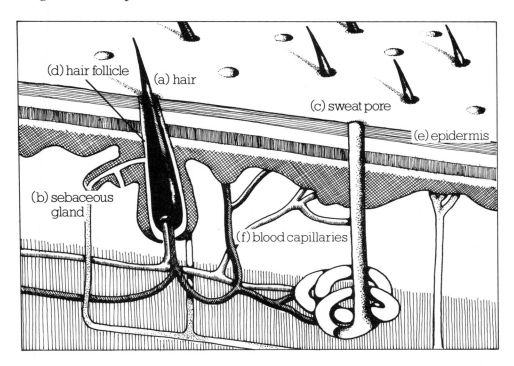

All skins produce their own moisturizers. Our bodies are covered with small hairs (a) and every hair has its own oil gland (b), called the sebaceous gland which is designed to produce oil – called sebum – which keeps the hair supple. The activity of these little glands producing sebum can vary in different areas; for instance, they are more active down the centre of the face than on the cheeks. The water which mixes with the sebum comes from the sweat glands (c): these and the hair follicles (d) account for the openings in our skins. If the skin is oily, which means that it is producing a lot of sebum, the latter can lie on the surface of the skin and unless the skin is thoroughly clean, it will settle in the tops of the skin openings, where it goes brown on contact with the air. This is what is commonly known as a blackhead. If you do have blackheads, professional facials are the most effective way of dealing with them.

The reason an oily skin is more troubled by spots than a dry skin is simply that the excess of sebum which lies on the surface is susceptible to bacterial infection from such things as air and hands. Once the skin openings get blocked they are more likely to form spots.

Obviously if you have a dry skin there is much less of this sebum on the skin surface, and therefore you are unlikely to be troubled by blackheads. You will notice also that the texture of your skin is different from that of an oily-skinned person in that the pores are much less noticeable. You will find however, that your skin normally gets dry because it lacks sufficient of the natural moisturizers, sebum and water.

The other important difference between dry skins and oily skins is their reaction to sunlight. Oily skins have plenty of brown pigment – called melanin – which comes to the surface to protect the skin. Fair, dry skins have much less of this protective pigment and what there is comes to the surface unevenly and slowly in the form of freckles, which make the skin much more inclined to burn.

Skin Types
In order to look after your skin it is important to know your skin type. Skins fall into four categories: dry, greasy, combination and problem. Although the standard test for diagnosing your skin type is not completely fool-proof, it may help you to decide which skin type applies to you.

Examine your face first thing in the morning – do make sure that you have cleaned it very thoroughly the night before – and standing in a good light wipe your face with a clean tissue, using half the double thickness. Then hold the tissue up to the light. If there are any transparent marks on the tissue these have been caused by oil from your skin. A greasy skin will show oil marks all over, a dry skin will show hardly any signs of transparency. Most people find that the oil only shows up when they apply the tissue to the centre of their face, and this indicates that they have a combination skin – that is dry on the cheeks and oily down the centre panel where most of the little oil-producing glands are clustered.

Problem skins are usually self-evident and prone to blemishes on the chin and sometimes on the forehead. The general texture of the skin is usually coarse-pored and prone to blackheads. Since this type of skin is usually caused by an imbalance of gland function, it is best to seek professional advice on the correct treatment.

Cleansing

The way you clean your face should be related to the type of skin you have. Soap and water is an effective way of cleaning the skin, and it is a method favoured by dermatologists. The important point to remember is that it is advisable to use a non-scented complexion soap, rather than the scented scum-forming soaps that you buy in supermarkets. Many of the latter are very alkaline, and since the skin's own moisture – a mixture of sebum and sweat referred to earlier – is acid, an alkaline soap can upset the natural acid balance of the skin. It is this acid balance which is often referred to in beauty language as the skin's "acid mantle", or in more scientific terms as the pH of the skin.

Many of the newest of the dermatologically formulated skin-care ranges such as Clinique and more recently Erno Lazlo promote the use of soap and water washing rather than the cream, cleanse and tone routine, which has been the established idea for so long. My belief is that if your skin feels comfortable with soap and water washing it is a perfectly acceptable way of cleansing the face, but in many ways I think that anyone with a dry skin is better off using one of the new water soluble cosmetic washing creams and lotions, such as Max Factor's Geminesse Cream and Water Cleanser or Revlon's Moon Drops Gentle Action Washing Cleanser. To my mind they combine the best of both methods. These washing creams and lotions have the advantage of being formulated by cosmetic chemists and have a proper acid-alkaline balance, which makes them much kinder to the skin.

The traditional way of cleaning your skin, which was recommended by most beauty writers for years, is to use cleansing cream or milk. For anyone who wears make-up it is one of the best ways of cleansing the face. The cream or milk blends with the oils in cosmetics and makes removal easier. This is in fact the method I use for cleansing my face, but the method you use is very much a matter of personal opinion and I recommend that people follow the method they find most comfortable.

Generally speaking I do not feel that toners are a necessary part of today's cleansing routine. Alcohol toners were really introduced by cosmetic houses to counteract the oiliness of the early cream cleansers and the slightly sticky feeling women noticed in contrast to the freshness of soap and water. Too many women are still using harsh alcohol toners too freely on their skins. Many toners contain a high proportion of alcohol, and although they give a fresh tingly feeling to the skin which many women love and feel is doing

DRY	OILY	DUAL	PROBLEM
flaky patches — poor oil flow — delicate blood vessels —	surplus oil — blackheads & open pores sluggish blood vessels —	CHEEKS — Dry skin reaction CENTRE PANEL — Oily skin reaction	blackheads turning to spots bacterial infection — imbalance of gland function
creamy cleansers mild milks cosmetic washing cream or lotion (Ponds Cleansing Cream) (Payot Golden Rays) (Swedish Formula Cleansing Lotion)	mild non-scented soap, or astringent milk cosmetic washing cream or lotion (Simple Soap) (Anne French Cleansing Milk) (Mary Quant Come Clean Cleanser)	cosmetic washing cream or lotion soap or cleansing milk (Revlon Moondrops Deep Action Cleanser) (Neutrogena Soap) (Innoxa Cleansing Milk)	medicated pore lotion soap or wash (Charles of the Ritz Special Lotion) (Helena Rubinstein Bio Clear Wash) (Innoxa 41 Skin Shampoo)
non-alcohol toner cream face mask (Lancôme Tonic Douceur) (Elizabeth Arden Orange Mask)	astringent or pore lotion pore grains — clay-type face mask (Payot Lotion No.6) (Katherine Corbett Open Pore Lotion) (Helena Rubinstein Beauty Washing Grains) (Innoxa White Mask)	mild astring. toner–cheeks pore lotion–centre panel mild mask–cheeks astringent mask–centre p. (Lemon Delph Skin Freshener) (Boots No.7 Protein Enriched Mask) (Rimmel Oatmeal Beauty Pack)	medicated pore lotion — medicated mask (Helena Rubinstein Bio Clear Pore Lotion) (Innoxa Face Mask 41)
Protective daytime moisturizer — oil based conditioning night cream (Oil of Ulay) (Boots No.7 moisture cream)	light greaseless day moisturizer non oily pH balanced greaseless night conditioning cream (Almay Blotting Base) (Guerlain Emulsion pH 5.5)	alternate a protective moisturizing cream with greaseless moisturizer (Nivea Cream) (Roc Moisturizer for Mixed Skin)	(Payot Paté Grise) (Orlane Crème Active) medicated cream — anti-biotic treatment cream
almond and olive oil camomile and elderflower egg yolk and honey	yarrow egg white lemon cucumber juice	brewers yeast and milk cider vinegar elderflower	lemon oatmeal sea salt yarrow

	DRY	OILY	DUAL
CHARACTERISTICS	tendency to wrinkles particularly round eyes broken veins —	coarse pored — sallowness	wrinkling and veins on cheeks open pores round nose —
CLEANSING 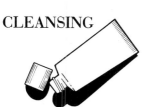	 rich cleansing milk or cream (Orlane Lacta Creme) (Max Factor Satin Flow)	cosmetic washing cream or lotion or mild soap (Geminesse Cream & Water Cleanser) (Roc Savon Surgras)	cleansing milk cosmetic wash 2 or 3 times a week (Almay Deep Mist Cleansing Lotion (Revlon Moondrops Deep Action Cleanser)
TONING 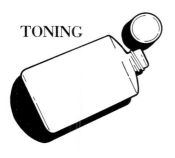	diluted non-alcohol toner or mineral water (Elizabeth Arden non-alcohol Skin Tonic) (Evian Brumisateur)	alcohol toner — pore grains — clay mask — (Helena Rubinstein Beauty Washing Grains) (Max Factor Astringent) (Orlane Masque Bleu)	non-alcohol toner — peel off gel mask (Cyclax Flower Balm) (Helena Rubinstein Brush-on Peel-off Mask)
NOURISHING 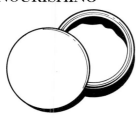	oil based day cream — rich night cream with active ingredients — eye and throat creams (Lancôme Hydrix) (Eterna 27 Night Cream) (Payot Eye Cream) (Orlane Oryane)	Eye cream greaseless pH balanced cream anti-blackhead cream (Clarins Eye Gel) (Charles of the Ritz Special Cream) (Guerlain Emulsion pH 5.5)	alternate oil based moisture cream on cheeks with water based moisturizer down centre panel (Vichy Equalia) (Roc crème Hydratant for oily skin)
NATURAL REMEDIES	honey egg yolk camomile avocado	lime flowers egg white yarrow and lettuce	brewers yeast and milk buttermilk lemon cucumber juice

them good, in my opinion the alcohol merely dries and coarsens the surface layer of the skin. These alcohol toners and astringents are really only suitable for young skins that are inclined to be spotty. The alcohol helps to sterilize and clean the skin and is a drying agent for spots.

If you have a normal or dry skin, but like the freshness of a toner, use one which states on the label that it is alcohol free: use it after cleansing your face with milk or cream.

Moisturizing

Women often ask if it is necessary to spend money on moisturizers. But when you pause to consider what central heating and strong sunlight can do to a piece of furniture, you realize that your skin needs all the help it can get.

The basic purpose of moisturizing is to supplement the skin's own moisture and to prevent the skin from drying out. It is important to realize that our skins naturally dehydrate as we grow older. A baby's skin contains eighty per cent moisture, whereas the average adult's skin has less than half that amount.

Moisture-retaining products are probably the most important skin-care development in the last thirty years. They throw a light protective film over the skin, and because most of these products are emulsions containing water, they are light and non-sticky.

To achieve the best results, moisturizing should be a two-step routine – day and night. Daytime products are extra light and designed to go on underneath your make-up. They act as an invisible lining between your skin and cosmetics, preventing colour pigments from coarsening the skin. Night moisturizers are normally formulated to work harder and often contain special skin-caring ingredients that are designed to help prevent the formation of little lines and wrinkles.

As you get older you may find that you need to use a cream stronger than a moisturizer at night. There is a wide variety of skin treatment creams to choose from. Many of these have special ingredients, which are based on hormonal extracts, and they have various names such as collagen and placenta. The principle of using female hormones – oestrogen – and synthetic hormones to help smooth out wrinkles is based on the fact that women's skins traditionally look better during pregnancy, due to the fact that pregnancy raises the oestrogen level of the body. Controlled experiments on groups of women have proved that changes in the skin have resulted from regular applications of small doses of oestrogen, but this is only really noticeable in women over forty. Most experts agree that a young healthy woman, whose body is functioning normally, already has enough oestrogen circulating in her blood stream to keep her skin looking fresh and unlined, so that a hormone cream will do very little for her. There is virtually no point in using these products until you are over forty.

When I asked a leading dermatologist whether in his opinion there were any creams marketed that were effective in reversing the ageing process, the answer he gave me was: "Unfortunately human beings aren't slot machines and putting a therapeutic coin in the right slot does not always produce the expected results. The most difficult problem about treating the skin is the variation in tissue sensitivity between one patient and another. A dose which is sufficient to produce a good effect on one person may have no effect on the next." He also pointed out that creams that were sold without prescription had to be carefully controlled so that the amount of, say, hormonal ingredient was relatively small in order to avoid the possibility of any tiresome side effects. Of the so-called skin-rejuvenating creams on the market, he thought those which had a hormonal derivative were the type most likely to produce the best results in helping to plump out lines and wrinkles. Many of the other ingredients used by cosmetic chemists for treating the skin, such as mink oil, and even one which was being used for the treatment of arthritis, have been incorporated into skin creams purely as a result of chance observation. For example, it was noticed that the skin on the hands of some older laboratory workers had shown a dramatic improvement while using ingredients for making products which had nothing to do with the skin. So creams containing these ingredients were developed.

The most controversial developments have been those involving test-tube ingredients. Even though tests have shown that synthetically produced steroid-type hormones do not have the side effects of natural oestrogen, such as brown patches due to a breakdown in pigmentation, or irritation, herbalists still say that we do not know nearly enough about the long-term effects on our bodies to experiment with such products. One herbalist I know had a patient who was convinced that she got a headache whenever she used a certain bath product which was scented with a synthetic fragrance. As he pointed out, though every plant has a purpose, scientifically made copies are still an unknown quantity. We cannot always be certain what the long-term effect of some of the ingredients will be, even if in the short term products made by reputable companies do seem to produce results.

There is no doubt that skin benefits from a change of beauty products from time to time. Most experts agree that the skin becomes accustomed to any treatment you use on it for too long, no matter how good, and after a while stops responding the way it did at first. There is nothing to be gained from sticking doggedly to the same products, and you will often find that a new routine will show better results. This is why I often recommend clients who have been using science-based skin products to change to products that are based on natural properties such as plants and herbs. If you have used only herb-based products for a long time, a more scientific cream can often act as a shock treatment to a dull, lifeless-looking skin.

Neck and Eye Creams

People often ask why they need special creams for the skin around their eyes and for their necks. The answer is that you can make do with your treatment night cream and use it on your neck as well as your face, and most of today's products are light enough to put on the delicate skin around the eyes without pulling and stretching the skin. But in that case they may be too light to be really effective on the coarser skin of the neck. Eye creams are no longer confined to the night shift; many products are made to an especially light formula which means that they can also be worn under make-up during the day. Most neck creams, too, are different from face creams as they contain astringents as well as oils which help to tone and give a smoother texture to the skin. Neck and eye skin-care products are in the medium and expensive price ranges, particularly since they are mainly intended for use by women over twenty-five.

Facials and Face Masks

You will see from the diagram of the skin that there is a layer of dry cuticle on the surface called the epidermis (e). If allowed to remain on the skin, it gives it a dry dehydrated look. One of the advantages of having a regular facial in a salon is that the face mask plus the stimulation caused by the massage helps to speed up the natural process by which these dead cells on the surface are removed and the reproductive cells are stimulated.

When talking to a group of women, I often ask how many of them buy the more expensive skin creams that are available on the market. Usually there are more than I expect there to be. I also ask for a show of hands on how many people have either had a facial in the last month or used a face mask, and I find that very few have done either. Personally I cannot see the point of spending large amounts of money on expensive skin creams, unless you also do something to prepare your skin and make it more receptive. A professional facial is one of the most valuable beauty treatments you can have. All facials include a face mask, which is the most effective method I know of cleansing the skin.

If you do not have a regular salon facial it is a good idea to use a face mask once a week. Nowadays there are face masks that are suitable for all types of skin. As well as the old style clay-type masks which left the skin feeling rather tight and were really only suitable for toning and purifying an oily skin, there are now milder gel masks which contain vegetable enzymes that absorb dead cuticle without drying the skin, and these are suitable for even the most delicate complexion. For home use there are three types of mask:

Clay, which is most suitable for oily skins
Cream, which is most suitable for dry skins
Gel, which is most suitable for normal to dry skins.

One of the advantages of the gel masks is that they peel off and do not need to be washed off in the same way that you have to remove a thick clay-type preparation. Cream masks are a milder version of the old-fashioned clay products and are therefore much less drying. Some set more firmly than others, but all are non-drying to the skin.

Broken Veins
These are little blood capillaries, which are shown on the skin diagram (f). Anyone who is a fair Nordic skin type will notice that the veins on her cheeks are much closer to the surface of the skin than those of people with coarser oilier skins which are inclined to be sallow. One of the reasons the latter develop a tan easily is that their capillaries are more protected and they do not dilate with the heat of the sun. They do not redden the surface skin as quickly as someone whose skin is very fine-textured. One of the real problems for a fair skin is to give adequate protection to these little blood capillaries which dilate in a warm temperature and contract in the cold.

When you are young the walls of these little capillaries are quite elastic, but with the natural ageing process they lose their elasticity, and if constantly bombarded with extremes of temperature such as hot sun or cold winds, or harsh alcohol toners, they are inclined to break, and you get little tracings of red veins appearing on the cheeks. One of the best reasons for wearing foundation, particularly one that contains moisturizing ingredients, is that it acts as a natural protection for the skin against the damaging effects of sunlight on the veins.

Doing It Yourself
Beauty is traditionally a do-it-yourself business, and in fact most salon treatments are based on home remedies, particularly face packs.

There are many books devoted to giving herbal recipes, if that is your overriding interest in beauty. But if like me you are interested in one or two simple recipes which you can use to give yourself a simple easy treatment at home, here are one or two suggestions.

My favourite home-made mask, which I find easy to make and effective in clearing the skin, is made by mixing wheat germ with a little milk.

For natural skin peeling I put a light film of vegetable or nut oil on my face with a few drops of warm water and pure lemon juice. I then wait a few minutes and before the mixture dries rub it off with my fingers.

As a refreshing face toner, try cider vinegar applied to your face with cotton wool: also use it in your bath to counteract the alkalinity of soap.

There are, of course, plenty of women who enjoy using fresh vegetables and fruits to make exotic natural skin treatments, and who will sit patiently with cucumber and honey on their faces, but I find that this tends to take up a lot of time and that I get just as good, if not better results with manufactured products, which have been professionally formulated. Such products always have good consistency, which I find difficult to achieve in home-made mixtures, added to the fact that they will not go rancid if not used up immediately.

Allergies

A favourite argument which many people use to support their use of natural products is that they feel their skin is less likely to have an allergic reaction to them. There is no doubt that the incidence of allergic reaction to cosmetics has increased considerably in the last fifteen years. The cause, in my opinion, is not as some women like to think due to the development of scientifically formulated cosmetic products: it owes much more to the increased pollution of the atmosphere, and more particularly to the increasing habit of manufacturers putting scent in almost every household product you can think of, such as furniture polish, detergents and air fresheners. Many people are also unknowingly sensitive to the nickel which is used in so many clothing fasteners: the irritant can easily be transferred to your face and neck.

There are about sixty known cosmetic irritants, and many of these will be found in the ingredients of natural products. They include lanolin, bees wax, cocoa butter, corn starch, rice starch, almond oil, boric acid and honey, to mention only a few, and this does not include most perfumes. The problem is that all sixty substances are perfectly pure and absolutely innocuous on the majority of skins, but on yours they may unfortunately spell trouble.

Luckily, it is now known that many potential irritants that used to be in cosmetics are not essential; for instance, it is not necessary for a lipstick to be scented. The scent does nothing to improve the colour, which after all is what ninety per cent of women want from a lipstick. Many other superfluous ingredients which used to be added to products for the sake of improving texture and feel have since been screened out, when they have been found to cause irritant reactions.

The answer to many people who find they are allergic to most cosmetics is to try one of the hypo-allergenic ranges, but remember there is always someone in the world on whose skin even hypo-allergenic and non-irritant ranges will cause irritation. The word "hypo-allergenic" means that any known irritants have been kept out of the formulation of these products, particularly scents, and that they have been exhaustively tested. In fact they are far less likely to cause an allergic reaction than are many of the home remedies we make ourselves using natural products.

One example of the contradiction that exists as to what are and are not irritant products is the popular use of baby lotion which, "because it's pure enough for babies, it must be pure enough for me". But there are women who have found that they developed an allergic reaction after using it, mainly because it contains an antiseptic, which in some very rare cases can make the skin sensitive.

One of the problems about allergies is discovering exactly what it is that you react to. If you have a reaction, which you think has been caused by an ingredient in some cosmetic you have used, it is worth taking a little trouble to try to discover whether you have correctly identified which product is actually the culprit, particularly if it cost you quite a lot of money. Try doing a simple test by putting a trace of the product on your neck with a dampened plaster over it, and leave it for twenty-four hours. If there is any redness on the spot, or you get any irritation, you will know that this is the product. If there are no signs, then carry on eliminating the other products you use until you find the one at fault.

SALON BEAUTY

Salons were originally started for the rich and leisured classes. There is still no doubt that an hour or two spent in a beauty salon is one of the most relaxing and pleasant ways of passing an afternoon; but with the rise in people's standards of living and the increase in the type of treatments that salons now provide, many of them due to the development of beauty machinery, people are beginning to realize that salons are no longer only for the rich.

Women who have never been to a salon before tend to be very shy about coming in for the first time – often I think because salons tend to make themselves a little forbidding and salon owners are inclined to encourage their girls to be a little too "expert" in their attitude to clients. I firmly believe there is no point, and in fact considerable damage all round, if you make a woman who has come into your salon for the first time feel that she knows nothing about beauty and is a fool because she does not. As discussed in the first chapter beauty is like a magic circle, and the more you know the more you are in a position to learn; it is those outside the circle who are in such a difficult position. It is salon owners and their girls who can help them break in.

I have found that quite often it is the problem of superfluous hair that will get many not very beauty-conscious women into a salon for the first time. Most women find that as they reach their mid-forties hairs start sprouting in all sorts of unwanted places, often on their upper lips – in just the place where many years earlier they used to smile at their elderly spinster aunt's moustache. There are of course a number of ways of removing such hair, but none as effectively as electrolysis, and this almost certainly means a visit to a salon.

Often after one or two visits, these women discover the wider pleasures of beauty salons. Of course life can be lived perfectly adequately without ever going near a beauty salon. This is particularly true for Englishwomen whose fair, dry, fine-pored skins seldom give much trouble, especially when they are young; this is very much in contrast to continental women who usually find they have to visit a beauty expert regularly: their oily skins need constant attention to control the flow of oil and keep them clean. Their skins are naturally oilier, and frequently aggravated by rich, oily food.

This is one of the many reasons why beauty experts and salons have for

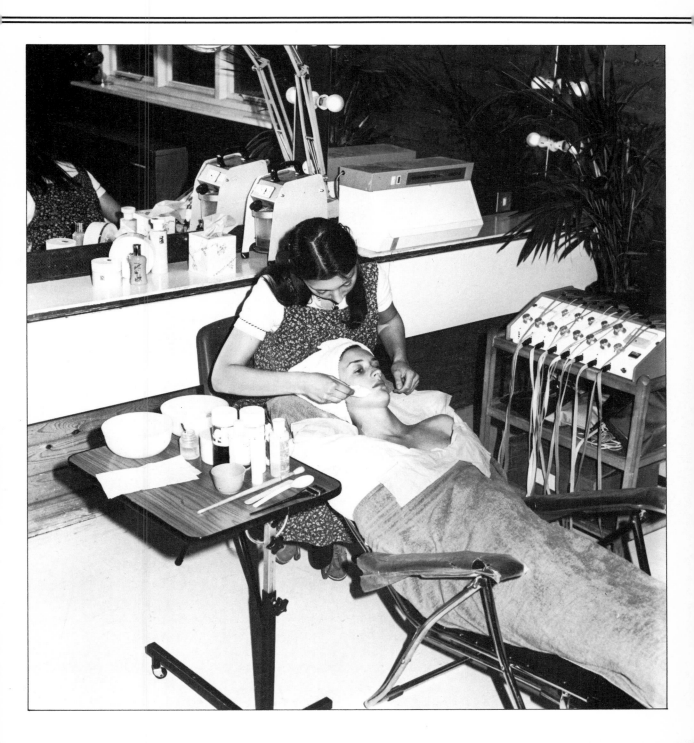

so many years been part of the continental scene. Many of the most successful beauticians have come from Central Europe: quite apart from universally recognized names such as Helena Rubinstein, Max Factor and more recently Dr Erno Lazlo, who dominated New York in the sixties, many of the leading private therapists like Maria Hornes, Helen Harnik and Countess Csaky have introduced to this country the techniques and recipes they learnt in Europe. In fact, the tradition of the continental salon is one almost exclusively of skin care and has little to do with make-up. The idea of combining a facial with make-up is very much an American one, and one which I disapprove of.

There are in fact many reasons why a visit to a beauty salon is worthwhile. In today's changing world, many women find themselves leading lonely lives and are surprisingly cut off from other people. A number of psychologists have told me that a lot of women lack sufficient physical contact, and that the contact they get in a beauty treatment can be very therapeutic – so much so, that in a number of psychiatric hospitals and homes, patients are actively encouraged to have facials.

Getting the best out of a beauty treatment means finding the right specialist or salon to suit your individual requirements. To start with there is the private therapist who gives a very personal kind of service and usually works on her own, sometimes in her home, offering her own skills rather on the same lines as a private dressmaker. She is usually the carefully guarded secret of her clientele, and although she may make a few specialized skin creams and lotions she does not market them. At the other end of the scale there are the Elizabeth Arden salons where you can enjoy every kind of treatment for hair and body, although with present day labour intensive costs, Arden is the only remaining internationally named salon in this country.

The right way to choose one of these individual beauty specialists who operate in the continental tradition is to discover what aspect of skin care they specialize in. If your problem is acne there are experts who have treatments for this condition and tackle the problem more like a dermatologist than a beautician. One of the best known of these is Julie Hacker, an English specialist who has been trained in the continental tradition. She gives treatments which consist of using oxygen to purify the skin and reckons there is no substitute for clearing the skin by hand. As long as the impurities are there, they are bound to erupt sooner or later, so you have to tackle the problem by extraction rather than simply cleaning the surface of the skin. She and Hungarian specialists such as Agnes Balint and Countess Csaky all have their own special remedies for skin problems. In fact their skills are the power behind some of the world's famous faces and their names are the closely guarded secrets of their clients. "My dear," said the beautiful woman draped in sables at the airport, "my skin looked so awful until I went to see . . .", and she lowers her voice into a tantalizing whisper. This is one reason why the names of specialists are not well known and the essence of their success is the exclusivity of their clientele. If you think that it is all a great deal of hocus pokus which no sane person would believe in, one of the most celebrated of the specialists, a certain Madame Lubatti, used natural cultures made from bacteria which came from the walls of Egyptian tombs which she had prepared especially to suit individual skins. One of her most regular clients was in fact a member of the Royal Family.

Countess Csaky is the well-kept secret of many of today's celebrated beauties. Her patients fly to London to see her from all over Europe. In fact there are several who come over regularly from Paris to have a treatment and return the same day. She works with her assistant in her Mayfair flat and her clients have to give plenty of notice in making appointments. She feels that the individual attention that the private specialist gives is really part of the treatment and makes the woman feel important. Many of her patients think that they should come to her more often, especially as they get older, but she always tries to persuade them that the skin is like a clock, which needs to be wound up, and as long as it has regular care it will keep in good condition.

Most of these specialists make their own lotions and creams rather than use the preparations that are available from the big manufacturers. As one of them explained to me, "I make all my own preparations because I like to know what's in a cream before I recommend it." However this means that whilst you can get good all-round advice and products on skin care, none of these ladies is really equipped to do modern up-to-date make-ups because they do not have the products that are needed for the contemporary face. In a way this is no bad thing since it is not sensible to have a make-up directly following a facial treatment; the skin is over-stimulated and needs time to settle down before applying much make-up.

In this country some of the most luxurious salons today are to be found in the big department stores which are usually well patronized by account customers who can put this luxury down on the household bill. For most people, the atmosphere of luxury and the high ratio of staff to client encourages them to feel pampered.

Often women are confused by the names given to various establishments. Many beauty therapists use the word "clinic" because they specialize in skin care, slimming and hair removal, but in my view this can be off-putting and creates too formal and medical an atmosphere; and because many young beauticians are nurses *manqués* who like to rustle round in white uniforms the whole feeling can become rather forbidding. I prefer the idea of a beauty shop or beauty salon where the atmosphere is more informal and in my view more suited to the Englishwoman's more lighthearted approach to beauty. Though if you need a highly specialized treatment, such as is needed if you have a serious superfluous hair problem, I should recommend you to go to a therapist who works on her clients herself, rather than to one who employs beauticians. The specialist has usually spent a lifetime developing and improving her techniques and you will get the benefit of her very specialized knowledge.

That is not to say that larger salons do not have their place. As someone who runs two, I very much believe that they do. To begin with, they can normally afford to have a wide range of machinery and equipment; and in the last ten years beauty machinery really has made great strides forward.

I also firmly believe that you will get much better and more informed help in make-up techniques and skin care from a salon which employs a number of girls, rather than just one or two. It is important that the girls can see each other working on clients' make-up, exchange ideas, discuss the new looks and techniques amongst each other, if they are going to stay right up to date.

Make-up is an area where many salons tend to be a bit dated. For example, they give clients a make-up following a facial, while they are still lying down. It is in fact impossible to put a contemporary make-up on to a woman's face when she is lying down and still feeling dozy after a relaxing treatment. Apart from a little foundation, powder, mascara and lipstick, there is no way you can apply a full make-up to a woman's face unless she is sitting facing a mirror. In any case the disadvantage of the old system of having a girl to put on your make-up after a facial was that when you got home you wondered what she had used and how it had been done. The sadness about the system is that the very people who are most qualified to advise you on skin-care products and make-up are in fact beauticians who work in salons. They are trained beauticians and have undergone a strenuous training, unlike the consultants in stores who are sales girls who have usually been given a few days' beauty training. In fact many women are not aware that the so-called experts and consultants in the cosmetic departments of stores are paid by the manufacturers and not the stores. Their advice is seldom impartial, as they are paid commission on sales and often trained to sell "five" – that is five products to each customer.

The treatment girl in a salon is able to judge your sensitivity to skin products during the facial, but because most salons do not have money invested in skin-care preparations from the big manufacturers, she cannot help you to find the right products which are available at chemists and stores, and the same is true of make-up. If the salon sends you out looking stunning they may have used leading brands which they do not stock, and the chances are they will have to tell you to buy them at your local store.

Beauty salons are a high risk business; it takes little imagination to realize that women can be physically damaged in a salon, so the insurers will only cover fully-qualified staff who know what they are talking about in all aspects of beauty. As on the continent, there is a strong move to ensure that any premises offering treatments only employ girls who have reached a professional standard in their work. One reason for this is that the state is becoming more involved with beauty than many people realize; this is in line with a trend which is far more developed on the continent than in this country. In Switzerland, for example, a beautician has to take a national examination, which is supervised by the state. In this country the local council has the power to control the giving of many body treatments to members of the public. In most major cities and some rural areas you have to be licensed if you wish to run a beauty salon, and the council ensures that the beauticians employed are properly trained by recognized schools. Most of these schools insist on at least a six-month course as a minimum, and it is comforting to know that the girls so trained have to achieve a considerable proficiency in subjects such as anatomy and physiology, electricity and chemistry. So the girl who is giving you a body massage does at least know which muscles she is working on.

In anatomy and physiology girls should achieve a good nursing standard, and it is interesting to note that in this respect we are considerably ahead of salons in America. For instance, one of my girls with top international qualifications went to work on the west coast of America three years ago, and was startled to find herself working amongst girls who had been picked up by the salon owner and taught a few basic facial massage movements. They were called beauticians!

Although I often feel that we have a surplus of bureaucracy, any woman visiting a salon in London will find it reassuring to know we have to submit a list of all the girls we employ, their qualifications, and even a certificate from an electrician to say the equipment has been inspected and is in full working order. Incidentally, I am often asked by my clients who have teenage sons suffering from acne if we can give their boys facials to clear up their spots. However, so strict are the by-laws that an establishment that is licensed for the treatment of women is not allowed to treat men as well, without separate facilities such as lavatories and changing rooms.

Salons now cover a wide range of treatments, and here is a guide to most of the ones which you will find offered in salons. Not all salons offer the whole range, and some prefer one type of treatment to another. But all the treatments mentioned have a very real purpose.

Electrolysis

This is the only really permanent method of removing hair, and it must be done by a skilled operator. She inserts a needle into the skin down to the root of the hair. A mild electric current is passed into the needle and cauterizes the root by cutting off the blood supply that feeds the hair. The more experienced your operator the more lasting the treatment, as she can adjust the strength of the current and the size of the needle she uses to give a maximum effectiveness with minimum discomfort. In my view salon electrolysists should be members of the Association of Electrolysists or the Institute of Electrolysists: the latter have the letters DRE after their names and are fully qualified to tackle medical hair problems such as hair down the neck and on the chest.

Electrolysis is neither cheap nor quick and most people find that they cannot have more than an hour's hair removal treatment at one sitting. For example, a fifty-year-old woman with a hair problem on her face will find that she probably needs two or three half-hour treatments to tidy up her upper lip, plus a subsequent quarter-hour check every now and then to tackle re-growth hairs that were still in the root when she had the original treatment.

Some women have a psychological reaction against electrolysis or find it too painful. For them there is a new alternative method, although I am doubtful if it is quite as permanent as electrolysis. It comprises electrical tweezers that grip the hair but do not touch the skin and the current is transferred down the hair shaft into the skin so that the hair lifts out. My experience is that this method can be effective in discouraging growth and is a very real alternative for those who for one reason or another find electrolysis too painful. The best-known version of this treatment is called Depilex and there are now experienced operators in many beauty salons all over the country. Because electrolysis and the electric tweezer method are slow and the cost high, these treatments are only really suitable for removing hairs on the face, though some women also use them to have the hair round the nipples removed.

Waxing

This is one of the oldest methods of removing hair, and was certainly practised by many early civilizations. It is possible to remove hairs by waxing at home, but the problems of heating the wax and then keeping it at a regular temperature can be difficult. Good salons are equipped to cope with all waxing; they have the latest waxing machines which thermostatically control the heat of the wax. They use special wax, a mixture of beeswax and resin, which is applied in strips and pulled off against the growth of the hair. A good and experienced salon waxer can make what is painful when inexpertly done, straightforward and simple.

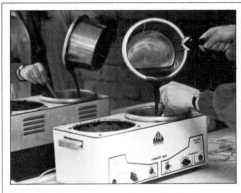

Wax for hair removal is melted down and kept warm ready for use. Talcum powder is rubbed on the leg.

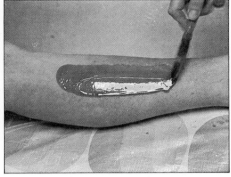

Wax is then applied in strips and spread in the opposite direction to the growth of the hair.

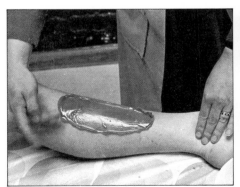

Wax is left to cool and the bottom edge is lifted to facilitate removal.

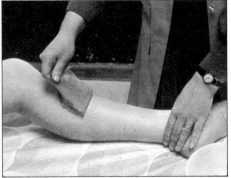

Wax is removed by stripping quickly against the growth of hair. The essence of good waxing is the speed of removal.

Waxing is an effective way of removing hairs from large areas of the body, particularly legs and the "bikini strip" in the groin. It lifts the hair from the root and normally when legs have been well waxed, they should not need re-waxing for about five to six weeks even in summer. Waxing can also be a useful way of removing hair from lips, particularly if you dislike electrolysis. At the Face Place, we have developed a method of shaping eyebrows with cold wax. We have found that we can get a better shape by using our method than you can by individual plucking.

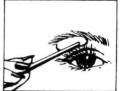 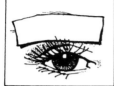 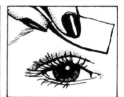 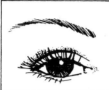

An effective alternative to plucking eyebrows is to wax them. Buy cold depilatory wax and apply underneath brows where stragglers grow.	Allow heat of skin to melt wax and spread thinly in an arc. Cut out a strip of material and place it over the wax. Rub it slightly so the material sticks to the wax.	Pick up a corner of the material furthest away from your nose and rip off quickly towards your nose. Always pull it in the opposite way to the way the hairs grow.	The skin under the brow is now free of hair. Pluck any remaining hair with tweezers. You always wax or pluck eyebrows from underneath, not above the brow.

Facials

Facials are one of the main activities of any salon. I also believe that they are an important part of any woman's beauty routine. When I first started the Face Place, we only sold cosmetics and gave advice about make-up and skin care. We soon found that neglected skin was a major problem for many women and it was this fact more than anything else which pushed us into giving treatments as well as advice.

I have discussed in the chapter on skin care the importance of cleansing your face. The point I want to make here is that many women find it impossible to cope with blackheads themselves, and many people allow the dry cuticle – little flakes of dead skin which are invisible to the naked eye – to remain on the surface of the skin giving it a dull dehydrated look. Men shave every day which is a natural cuticle removing – or exfoliating – process. By scraping their faces with a razor they remove dead surface skin, but the only way that we women can do the same thing is either by having a facial or by using a face mask regularly at home.

The use of a face mask is an important part of the facial process. I believe it is pointless to spend a lot of money on expensive night creams and moisturizers, unless you also do something to prepare the skin so that they are properly absorbed. Regular facials will do this as well as stimulate the circulation to nourish the skin from inside by face massage, and remove blackheads – after the pores of the skin have been relaxed by steaming. A good well-executed facial can be pleasurable and relaxing, and is one of the best ways of keeping your skin in good condition.

It is, of course, possible to give yourself a facial at home but you have to be very strong-minded about ignoring all interruptions such as the telephone or front doorbell and you will miss the pleasure of the relaxed feeling you get from a salon facial.

A major advance in facial treatments in the last forty years has been the development of electrical currents for increasing the effectiveness of a facial. Although galvanic treatments have been known and used for many years, recent technology has increased their scope considerably.

Normally it is one of the skin's functions to prevent penetration of substances on its surface. Face creams, in fact, act mainly as sealers, helping the skin to retain its natural moisture. However, the use of a very mild electrical current, passed through special active substances called ions, allows treatment serums to achieve a greater absorption into the skin. This deeper absorption helps to nourish the lower levels of the skin and speed up its reproductive processes, so combating wrinkles and the ageing effect of sunlight. In fact the effects of the sun and of the ultra-violet rays are now reckoned by dermatologists to be the major factor in the ageing process. Because the sun thickens the outer layers of the skin and so lessens its ability to absorb creams, it requires more than a simple face massage to penetrate the lower levels of the skin.

One of the most popular uses of a galvanic current is a method called Cathiodermie, which applies the current to the skin through small metal rollers.

Another variation of the use of electrical current is known as descincrustation and is used for treating greasy skin which is one of the most common skin problems. Once again liquids are passed into the skin by means of galvanic current, but through a tweezer-like electrode instead of rollers, around which cotton wool dampened in a saline solution has been wrapped. This causes a chemical reaction within the oil glands and helps to dry out superfluous grease.

Treatments using galvanic current are usually followed by a second form of electrical stimulation called high frequency. This gives a mild tingling

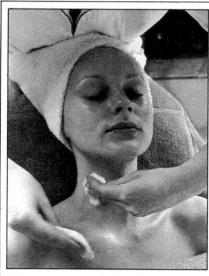

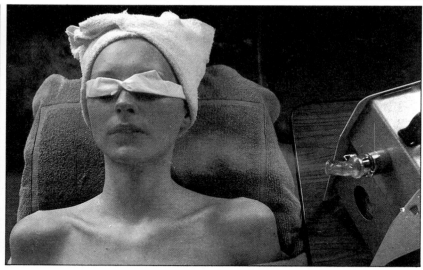

A facial starts with face and neck cleansing using cream or lotion: skin is then examined for blocked pores and blackheads.

The face is then steamed which helps to relax the pores and assist in the clearing of blackheads. The steamer incorporates an ultra violet unit that produces a fine ozone vapour that purifies and helps to promote healing for spots and blemishes.

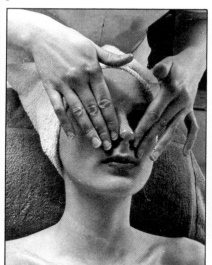

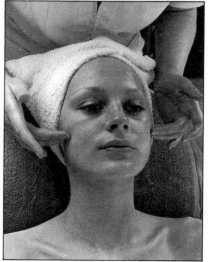

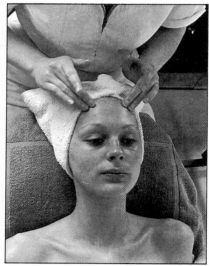

Attention is paid to removing blackheads from the centre of the face where oil-producing sebaceous glands are active.

Face and neck are then gently massaged to stimulate circulation and to reduce puffiness caused by water retention.

The massage ends at the forehead. A good facial massage can be relaxing and clients often fall asleep at the end.

sensation and it is applied to the skin through gauze: this helps to close the pores, leaving the skin toned up and looking clearer.

The use of electrical stimulation for treating different skin conditions in the hands of a skilled beauty therapist can do a great deal to clear problems such as acne, and clients who have this type of treatment regularly find that the wrinkle-smoothing and deep-cleansing effects are excellent.

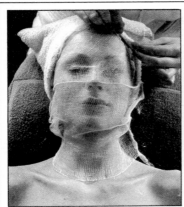 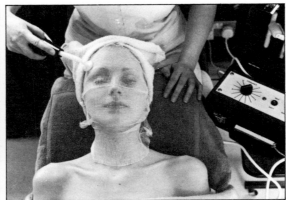

Facials incorporating an electrical current are particularly effective for deep-cleansing the skin and extracting impurities. Here gauze is used to cover the face so that the electrical applicator can glide smoothly over the skin.
One of the most successful of these electrical facial treatments is known as Cathiodermie.

I find that many women have the misconception that salon facials are a luxurious way of passing the time for rich women. Today, when most of us spend so much time rushing around, the experience of an hour's facial can be not only relaxing but therapeutic. In fact, the value you get for the price of an hour's facial is remarkable, taking into account the skill required to be a good beautician.

One of the advantages of having a facial from a trained beautician is that, once she has had the opportunity to examine your skin closely and to see how it reacts, she can give you accurate advice on what products are best suited to it. This is likely to be considerably more accurate than the advice given by a sales consultant.

Herbal Skin Peeling
This has particular use for people whose skin used to be oily, and who have been left with scar tissue from bad acne. It also helps to refine a coarse-

pored skin. Skin peeling works in much the same way as sunburn. In an extreme form it is usually only done by a plastic surgeon. A chemical is used to "burn off" the surface layer of the skin causing redness, dryness and blistering. This extreme form of skin peeling is called dermabrasion because it is sometimes combined with the use of an abrasive skin plane. This is dealt with more fully in the chapter on plastic surgery.

Salon skin peeling is a much milder version of the surgical peel. Instead of chemicals, herbal remedies are used which cause minor surface dryness. The beauty specialist does a special type of abrasive massage, which helps to remove dead cuticle, and leaves the skin looking clearer and smoother. Obviously this milder treatment does not have such dramatic skin clearing results, but if given on a regular basis can do a great deal to improve the texture of a coarse-pored skin.

Aromatherapy

An increasingly popular type of face treatment today is called aromatherapy, and it is based on the use of essential oils. These essential oils are found in the root bark leaves of flowers and of aromatic plants such as bergamot, lavender, rosemary, camomile and thyme. The oils are extracted from the plant by distillation, and practitioners of aromatherapy claim that because these oils contain the essential life force they can be transmitted into the human organism by massage.

Various types of massage are used and most of the diagnostic work which is a feature of your first aromatherapy treatment is done on your back. The aromatherapist works on nerves and muscles following the energy pathways of the body in much the same way as a practitioner in acupuncture. Oils are individually prescribed in order to promote health and well-being to the body. In my view this is a very relaxing form of beauty treatment and since it was introduced into this country by Madame Maury in the fifties, it has become increasingly popular.

I do not feel, however, that most of the aromatherapy treatments given in the salons today have much to do with the original healing, health promoting concept of this treatment. The only exceptions are the treatments given by two specialists who used to work with the legendary Madam Maury when she was living in this country in the late fifties and who had specialized in aromatherapy for many years.

Micheline Arcier is French and Dany Ryman English, and both have small exclusive salons in London where they do this work. Madame Arcier worked as a beautician for several years in France before she met Madame Maury. She discovered that, "When I worked with essential oils extracted from plants they seemed to have very swift healing powers on the skin. Especially when used in conjunction with massage, the vegetable hormones seemed to increase the growth of new vigorous skin cells." Both Micheline and Dany say that they can tell a great deal about a person's health from the face. For instance deep nose to mouth lines are often a sign of stomach trouble and any slight puffiness particularly under the eyes shows a tendency to water retention. "Aromatherapy treatments have a wonderful psychological effect," says Dany. "By treating the whole organism you discover which group of muscles want relaxing. Once you have broken down the physical tension, people also feel mentally relieved. My clients just relax and start talking about all their problems."

Eyelash Dyeing

If your lashes are scanty or really fair so that you wake up in the morning looking like an albino rabbit, you should consider having an eyelash dye. The process is the same as tinting your hair, but with modern vegetable dyes it is now completely safe. The colour stays in your lashes until they fall out in the normal way and are replaced by fair lashes, which usually takes about four to five weeks. In the old days eyelash dyeing or lash tinting was given the status of a full treatment in most beauty salons. The colour was applied to the lashes while you lay back on a facial couch in a darkened treatment room. I have found that this operation can be speeded up and at

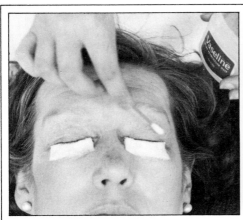

Small damp cotton wool pads are placed under the eyes to keep the dye away from the skin.

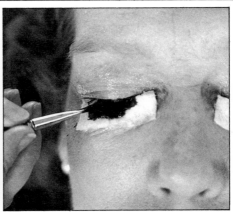

Lash dye is then applied with a brush first to bottom lashes and then to top lashes.

the Face Place we do lash dyes sitting up in the salon, so that the whole process only takes fifteen minutes and is much less of a performance.

The most usual colour is a mixture of brown and black; for a darker effect, blue mixed with black can be very effective.

Lash dyeing is not a total substitute for wearing mascara, although many women have it done for this reason. In my view mascara is still needed for evening as it helps to thicken up sparse looking lashes.

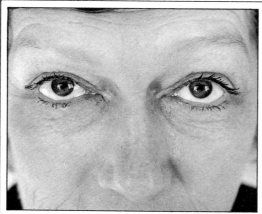

The development of vegetable dyes has changed eyelash dyeing in the last fifteen years from a difficult and risky treatment to an increasingly popular one in all beauty salons today. It is particularly useful to women with fair sandy lashes as it gives definition to the eyes and saves them from always having to worry about wearing mascara. An eyelash dye is completely water-proof and lasts for about five to six weeks until the lashes grow out. For evening it is often advisable to put mascara on top to get a thicker effect.

Sun-Lamp Treatments

These have been dealt with more fully in "Sun Looks". Most quartz solaria do not give you much colour, and exposure needs to be carefully timed. However, there are now sun beds where the lamp is incorporated into the bed that you lie on. These have effectively screened out most of the burning rays so that timing is not restricted, and with frequent use it is possible to develop a good colour. It is always best to apply sun-cream preparations before any form of ultra-violet lamp exposure, even though the manufacturers of the latest machines claim that this is not necessary.

Body Treatments

The introduction of slimming machines which are now widely available in the salons has meant that you can now concentrate on spot reducing, that is reducing selected areas of the body. Machines cannot help you to lose weight: only dieting can do that. But machines and other aids can help you to deal with inches. Women can often be slim and yet have large measurements on hips, bottom and thighs – a pear shape is sometimes reckoned to be a characteristic of Englishwomen's figures. Many women find that as they move into their forties, they develop hard localized lumpy fat around the hips. This condition is usually referred to as cellulite and neither dieting, careful eating nor even exercise will affect it. One of the characteristics is that the skin has an uneven, orange peel, pitted look, particularly when you pinch these areas. The unevenness is caused by fluid and toxic impurities which get trapped in the tissues, and only a very strong machine massage will really help to break up this lumpy looking fat.

One of the most effective salon treatments for cellulite is a suction cup massage machine. This works on a powerful air-pumping principle, and gives a very deep massage which breaks down the deposits of hard fat and redistributes them more evenly. The skin becomes smoother and less pitted looking. It is important to have these treatments close together – at least three times a week. Widely spaced single treatments do not achieve satisfactory results.

Once on a course of six treatments taken three times a week, you should notice a marked improvement to the texture of the skin in these areas, and my customers find that after the fourth treatment they can wear a pair of jeans that were too tight before they started. Because of the strong, rolling, kneading action of this type of massage, customers often find they get a bit of bruising; this will soon wear off. This type of concentrated treatment is only suitable for hard fat areas.

I find the Autoslim is one of the most effective of the various suction cup massage machines that are used in salons. Besides being extremely powerful, it operates automatically and can give a long sustained treatment, which really breaks down the cellulite.

The other main area for spot reducing is the waist-line and tummy, where women find the muscles have got slack after having had children. A muscle exercising machine such as Slendertone or Cellutron, which uses faradic current, is the best answer for those soft fat areas. Pads are applied to the motor points of the muscles and give gentle electrical stimulation. In this way, muscles get more exercise in twenty minutes than you could give them if you did press-ups every day for six months.

Vibratory massagers have now been perfected so that they simulate a strong hand massage, and they can be used for toning muscles, breaking down fatty deposits and helping to disperse fluid on either hard or soft fat areas. The most widely used of these machines is called a G5. This gives deep vibratory massage applied to the body through a variety of foam-padded massage heads, which are suitable for different areas.

Steam Baths and Saunas
There are a number of popular misconceptions about heat baths, such as

saunas, steam cabinet baths and Turkish baths. Because they are used extensively by jockeys to help them maintain a low weight, women think they are an answer to losing weight in a hurry.

It is perfectly true that if you induce perspiration by any of these methods you will lose a few pounds because of dehydration. However the results are in no way permanent and you tend to put back what you have lost as soon as you start to drink again – even by having a cup of tea. Each has advantages and disadvantages: saunas give a drier heat because the timber absorbs a lot of the moisture, but some people find them a little uncomfortable because the face and mouth are exposed to the heat. Steam cabinet baths make you perspire more quickly than a sauna. You sit boxed-up in padded comfort with steam circulating round your body on the same principle as you get with a Turkish Bath where you move from one hot room to another. I find steam cabinets very comfortable as your head is outside the cabinet and not exposed to the heat.

Frankly I think that these types of heat treatment do more to improve your skin than they do to improve your shape. Health hydros and beauty farms have a number of more sophisticated treatments, most of them involving the use of steam and water. In fact hydro-massage, where powerful jets of water are used to pummel the body and tone circulation, is normally standard equipment in most health farms. One version involves the use of high pressure hoses under water on soft muscle and tension spots; a German version of this treatment, which is often used, involves the application of contrasting temperatures of water to the pelvic area and feet. This constricts and dilates blood vessels in those areas in order to improve circulation.

This increasingly scientific approach to beauty is one of the main reasons for the ever-growing popularity of beauty salons today, and many women find that the discipline of a course of slimming involving regular visits to the salon for treatments is very helpful when they are trying to diet, particularly when they are doing it while feeding a family. The fact that they have spent money on a treatment can help to strengthen their resolution to stick to the rules.

Swedish Massage
Manual massage, usually called Swedish massage because most of the movements originated from that country where massage after a sauna is popular, is also a regular treatment in most salons and most beauticians have been taught their massage by a member of the Institute of Physiotherapists. Whilst a good masseuse can give you a massage which will help you to relax, she will not, in my view, have the strength to make a notice-

able difference to your measurements. If you are having manual massage, it is sensible to precede it with some form of heat treatment such as a sauna or steam cabinet bath, since the heat will relax your muscles and make the masseuse's job infinitely easier – and more comfortable for you. However, apart from stimulating the circulation which will improve your skin tone, and making it feel smoother by the use of oil, manual massage will not do much to improve your shape; this is the job of the machines.

Manicure and Pedicure
One of the best ways to be sure that hands, nails and feet always look well cared for is to have a professional manicure and pedicure. The main difference between cleaning and painting your own nails and having someone to do it for you is best described by the word "professional". A really skilled manicurist can make all the difference to the way your hands and feet look. It is of course perfectly possible to do an adequate job with a home manicure or pedicure, but a manicurist's skill is partly in the way she files your nails to compliment their shape, and in the painting, which because of years of experience always seems to last that bit longer without chipping. A professional manicure usually includes a massage to hands and feet, which can be very relaxing.

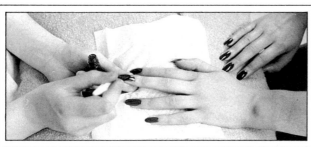

A professional manicure starts with your nails being shaped, then the cuticles are lifted with cream to release the acidity which causes them to stick to the nails: finally nails are painted with varnish.

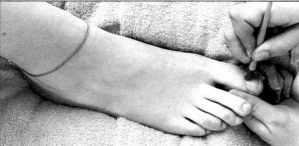

The same routine is followed as for hands. Strips of cotton wool are placed between the toes to keep them separated while the varnish is being applied and dries. If you are going to wear light strap sandals, a pedicure can improve the appearance of your feet.

If you have very neglected hands, try having a wax manicure. For this type of manicure warm paraffin wax is used, which unlike depilatory wax is not sticky. The wax is first painted on to the hands which are then wrapped in plastic and towels so that the warmth gets right into the hands. The hands then perspire, which helps to deep clean the skin and draw out the toxic impurities which are the main cause of stiffness, aches and pains.

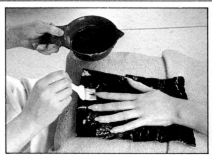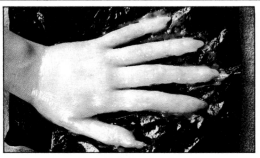

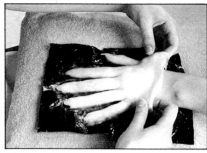

A good way of restoring softness to care-worn hands is to have a professional wax manicure. First, warm paraffin wax is spread over your hands, which are then wrapped in towels to keep in the heat. The warmth of the wax allows the skin to absorb the paraffin, which softens the skin. After twenty minutes the hands are unwrapped and the wax removed. This treatment is beneficial for arthritic or rheumatic hands.

Ear Piercing

There is good news for you, if you are one of those people who has not had her ears pierced because you think of all the horrors of the old methods such as the needle and cork, or feel that the more hygienic method with a local anaesthetic and surgical sleeper plugs is too much like an operation. There is a new painless method from America. It takes only five minutes and most women, having screwed up their courage for the operation, are amazed at the ease with which it is done. It involves a gun, rather like a stapling gun, and gold plated or real gold studs are used instead of sleepers. You keep them in for five weeks and wipe the lobes daily with surgical spirit, and after that time you can take them out and wear any other earrings. We do hundreds of ear piercings a year, and everyone is surprised how easy and simple it now is. It sounds too easy to be true; but it is.

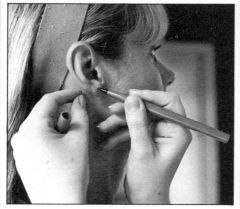

An antiseptic marker pen identifies where the ear is to be pierced.

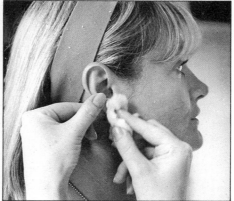

The lobe is then wiped with surgical spirit to guard against any infection.

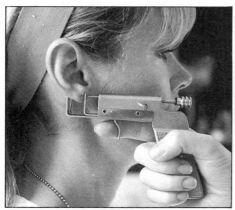

The special ear-piercing gun is placed against the mark on the ear and fired.

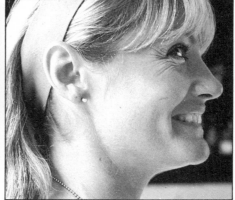

The ear is now pierced with the stud in place. It really is as simple as that.

MAKING FACES

As I have said in the first chapter, making up is in many ways like cooking: the more you know, the better you get at doing it, the more interested you become. The greatest enemy to making up is the attitude of mind which says what I cannot do well, I am better not doing at all. In fact, there is no real reason why everyone should not be good at applying make-up. Of course you need some skill, but the basic requirements are a knowledge of what is involved, practice and time. Paradoxically, as the final look has become more natural, making up well has involved more products and more skill. This is something which many people find hard to appreciate. Let me tell a story which illustrates the point. I well remember sitting in one of those fashionable restaurants in the King's Road, in the late sixties, with a young Australian business colleague of my husband. He was on his first trip to Europe. At the end of lunch he turned to me and said, "I can't get over how beautiful all these young girls are: so much prettier than our Australian girls with all their make-up." "But Martin," I said, "the girls are probably wearing twice as much make-up as the girls in Australia!" He found it hard to believe, but it was true.

In the thirties, when the artificial look with its whitish face was fashionable, making up was relatively easy. It is the striving for the natural look which has made the whole matter so much more complicated, and involved so many more products.

Make-up today is about making the best of your good features and hiding the bad, but the final effect must look natural. This means plenty of light and shade, involving both shiny and matt products. Whereas twenty years ago a well made-up face would have involved five products, today's natural face requires about ten. But one word of consolation for the faint-hearted: make-up is certainly one area of beauty which owes more to skill than money. Do not choose make-up products by price, choose them by colour and texture, though I should add that it is frequently the younger ranges like Boots No. 7 which have the most up-to-date colours. More about colour in chapter 7.

The two most important aspects in making up are first, knowing what products to use and choosing the right colours, and second, how to apply them.

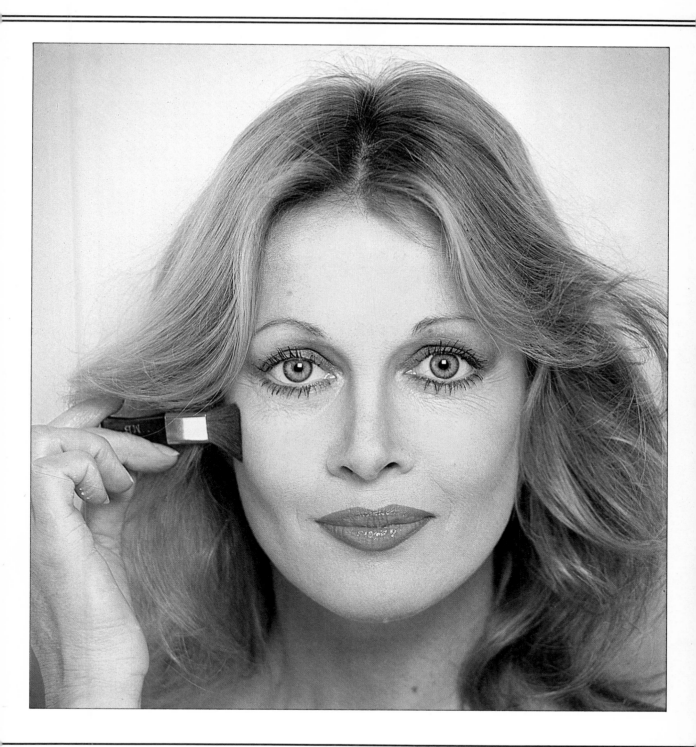

TOOLS FOR MAKING UP
Before you start on a make-up you need to have the right tools.

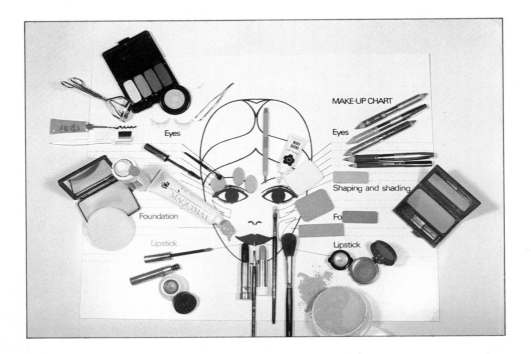

Cotton Wool and Cotton Buds
Cotton wool is the best aid for applying powder and all lotions. Cotton buds are critical to a good eye make-up, as they help to blend the colours together smoothly and evenly.

Foam Sponges
Small foam sponges, which can be bought from chemists, are the most professional way of making sure that your foundation has a smooth even finish. Even if you apply it with your fingertips, go over it with a sponge.

Brushes
Using brushes to apply make-up is a relatively new habit: they have always been used by theatre make-up artists, and are in fact essential equipment for the natural look. Without them you will find it difficult to achieve the refinement of shading that is required.

Brushes fall into two main categories: rouge mops and eye/lip brushes.

Rouge mops are large, generous brushes made of soft-textured but firm bristles. They are used for applying shaders and blushers. Eye and lip brushes have square or pointed heads. You need one square and two pointed brushes, one larger than the other. There are also eyebrow brushes which are shaped like small toothbrushes.

Tweezers
You will need a pair of tweezers for removing stray eyebrow hairs.

Sharpeners
Eye pencils need a special sharpener as their texture is too soft for them to be sharpened properly with a knife or a blade. Sharpeners are sold by a number of cosmetic manufacturers.

BASIC COLOURING

Moisturizer
Our make-up lesson starts with advice about finding the right moisturizer. Moisturizers have already been discussed in chapter 4: remember that the purpose of the moisturizer is to keep your skin feeling comfortable and to give it a good surface so that your foundation can go on smoothly and evenly.

Foundation
Choosing the right foundation is one of the most important aspects of making up well. Foundation is in fact the basis of the colour you wish to give to your face; over half the women I see make the mistake of thinking that their colour should come from their powder.

Foundations come in several forms: liquid, cream, cake, mousse and matt. The type you use depends on the effect you want.

Women with high colouring, that is apple-red cheeks and nose, need plenty of cover; for them the most suitable are a cream compact foundation or matt foundation.

Young skins can wear any type of foundation and for them it is basically a matter of using the one they find looks and feels best. Older women have less choice: if they have no colour to hide, the lighter the foundation they use the better, as heavy texture foundation shows up the wrinkles. For them, light aerosol mousses and liquids are ideal: most liquid foundations are fairly light, and the advantage of aerosol mousses is that they are invariably light, but sadly there are few brands on the market.

If you have an oily, coarse-pored skin, you need to be extra careful, as heavy foundations will give you an orange peel look. You will find that oil-free foundations are usually the best, as they are light and do not add more oil to an already oily skin. Oil-free foundations have names such as un-shine, pH fluid make-up or are just called oil-free.

You can also use foundation to give your skin a transparent tanned effect. For this you use one of the bronzing gels, or wash-off fake tans, described in detail in chapter 8.

The rules for finding the right foundation are simple, but frequently not followed and often misinterpreted.

1 Choose a beige or golden tint, rather than pink or peach: the latter colours invariably hot up and go orange after you have worn them for two or three hours. The first time you choose a beige or golden tone, you may be surprised that anything which looks so unappealing in the bottle could be the right colour for you. This is even truer when you choose make-up in the harsh strip-lighting favoured by stores. Blondes with fair, northern skin colouring need cool or fair beige tones with names such as bare beige, ivory beige or cream beige; darker faces should select warmer golden tones with shade names such as golden tan, toasty beige, or sun beige.

2 Remember that older skins have more pigment in them than younger skins, and if you are over forty and have always thought of yourself as the "fair peaches and cream type", years of exposure to sun will have altered your basic pigment. You should therefore wear the darker shades.

3 Never choose a foundation to brighten your skin. This is the function of the blushers; otherwise you will be like those elderly ladies who go around with bright pink faces that are a sharp contrast to the whiteness of their necks.

HIDING FLAWS

Although foundation will help to hide most of the flaws and imperfections of your skin, such as uneven pigment, redness, shadows under the eyes and even small pimples, it is sometimes a good idea to tackle these problems with a special flesh-tinted concealing cream, which goes on before your foundation. Although quite a number of women use medicated flesh-coloured cream sticks to cover up spots and even shadows under the eyes, there is a technique for using this type of cover-up cream which will give better results.

When it comes to hiding shadows under the eyes, it is absolutely vital to use the cover cream very sparingly, and it must be applied with a brush. Remember too, that the skin under the eyes is not flat and smooth-textured and that any of the cream that gets on to the puffier areas will merely make these look more noticeable. I tell my customers to keep a special make-up brush for applying this cream. When filling the brush with cream, it is important to use the back of your hand as a palette to thin out the amount you use, before applying it to the under-eye area; once you have loaded your brush you can keep it in a plastic bag on your dressing table, and you will find that you have enough on the brush for several applications. When applying the cream to the shadows under the eye, make sure that it only goes into the hollows, not on to any raised puffy areas; you can pat it gently with the finger to allow the warmth of the skin to melt it in smoothly. Never apply too much cream to the area or you will spoil the effect – several applications are better than one thick one – and never drag the delicate skin in this area by rubbing with your finger. Then you can take your brush and touch out some of the other little shadows on your face – in the same way that a professional make-up artist would do for a photographic make-up – nose to mouth lines, hollows at the corners of the mouth and on your chin can all be softened with this light concealing cream. The next step is to apply your foundation smoothly over the top.

Powder

Powder has probably changed its function in make-up more than any other product. Originally it was used for "powdering your nose", that is to prevent a shiny nose and face. Innovators like Harriet Hubbard Ayer, Helena Rubinstein and Max Factor then showed women that they could introduce colour to their faces by using pink or peach powders. Max Factor later introduced, from his experience in making up film stars in Hollywood, the idea of tinted greasepaint sticks, which were the forerunners of today's foundation.

For years after this, powder and foundation were colour matched. For instance, you bought Helena Rubinstein's Sport Light foundation with matching Sport Light powder. In the thirties Charles of the Ritz hit on the idea of producing "custom-blended" powder, that is powder hand-blended on the spot to match your complexion. There was a drawback about this powder: in order to achieve the right colour mix, the texture of the powder had to be thicker than milled powder. This meant that it tended to give a matt finish to the skin. One of the basic problems about tinted powder was that it gave a doll-like even finish to the skin, with no light and shade. This look was of course fashionable in the thirties and forties. But its artificiality meant that it could not last.

It is an interesting comment on changing fashions in social behaviour and attitudes that in the forties, when it was not done to make up in public, it was acceptable to powder your face. In fact the compacts of the day achieved the status of smart accessories. I remember compacts in the war with diamanté-studded RAF wings and regimental badges.

Max Factor's son achieved one of the biggest make-up booms of all time at the end of the war, by combining tinted foundation with tinted powder in one compact, and he called it Creme Puff. Its great appeal was that it gave instant coverage and hid all blemishes. But all tinted powders, particularly those which incorporated foundation, had the drawback that they tended to turn orange once you had worn them for a couple of hours. You found yourself with your face one colour and your neck another unless you took the powder right down your neck.

Today powder has a totally different function, and this is a point I find extremely difficult to communicate to women over forty. Its function today is nothing to do with adding colour; that, as I said earlier, is the purpose of foundation. Powder's function is to help to "set" your foundation, so that it does not rub off whenever you touch your face.

A lot of young women, particularly those who like the shiny look, tend to think that powder is old-fashioned and will date their make-up. I disagree. As long as the powder is truly colourless, and I agree that this is difficult to find, it will not take away the natural light and shade of your face, which is so important to a contemporary make-up. And if you want to keep the shine, use a translucent powder with a built-in shine ingredient. The reason it is so difficult to find a truly no-colour powder is partly that so many women still expect powder to have some colour in it, and partly because manufacturers colour it up with a touch of peach or pink for store lighting. For this reason, nearly all the leading make-up artists today use talcum powder. Unfortunately it is not applicable for everyday use, as you have to adjust your foundation colour to take into account the whiteness of talcum.

In choosing a powder, compare three or four so-called transparent powders, and take the one which looks the least coloured. The right powder to use for setting is loose powder. Compact powder should only be used for touching up during the day, as it tends to be over-compressed and gives too much blanket coverage.

There is skill in applying powder correctly. Always use cotton wool instead of a powder-puff because the grease from the old make-up will stick to the puff and destroy the consistency of the fresh powder. Press on the powder, rather than wiping it on to your face, so that it presses the foundation on to your skin. Any powder which is not absorbed into the foundation should be flicked off lightly with the clean side of the cotton wool.

SHAPING AND SHADING

Like so many make-up ideas, shaders originated in the theatre. A strong make-up was always necessary in the theatre, because the brightness of the footlights flattened an actress's features. The purpose of shaders is to hollow your cheeks and so define the bone structure of your face: a face with well-defined bone structure appears more interesting than a round chubby face.

When it comes to shaping and shading the face, many of my customers say that they find it very difficult to know what shape of face they have. One of the problems of make-up instruction in magazines is that much of the information is based on manuals written by professional artists, and these experts often vary their shading techniques to make a wide face look narrower and a long face look shorter. In my experience the amateur should not worry about diagnosing her face shape, but rather try to understand the basic principles of what she is trying to do, which is to introduce light, shade and glow to a flat canvas created by the foundation. Once you have mastered the basic techniques described in this chapter, you can then worry about how to adapt them to improve the shape of your face. One last warning while on this subject: do not be put off by the next magazine article you read, which may be crammed full of diagrams showing face shapes. As someone who has written beauty articles for many years, I know that art directors like to break up "boring" text with lots of illustrations which make for a much more interesting-looking page, but these illustrations are really only useful for professional models.

Another misconception about shaders is that you can shape and shade your face without using foundation. A customer often comes into my shop and says she wants to buy a new blusher. At which point one of my girls will ask her what foundation she is using. She will quite likely say that she never uses foundation, and is rather surprised to be told that she will not get much effect from a blusher unless she uses one. To get the best results from your blusher or shader it is necessary to use foundation to get rid of your own colour first, particularly that concentrated down the centre of your face around the nose, otherwise it will get in the way of the blusher.

Step-By-Step Make-Up

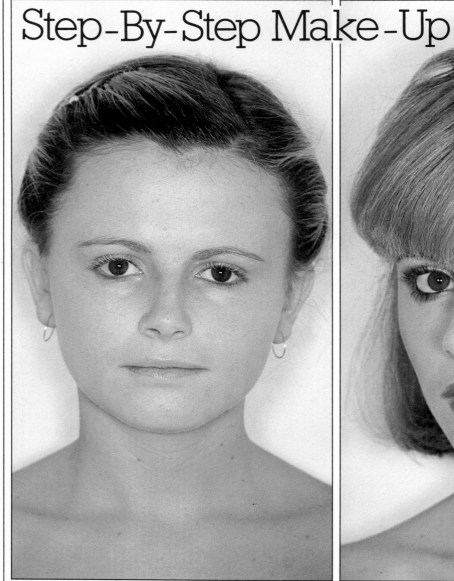
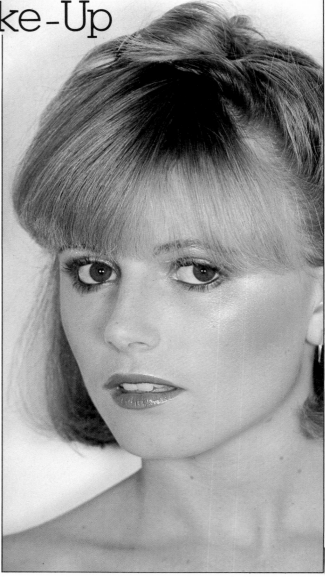

If you have ever doubted that the right make-up skilfully applied can improve on nature, take a look at these two pictures. They speak for themselves. Make-up helps all of us to emphasize our good points and play down the bad.

The pictures which follow show how to apply your make-up step by step to get the best effect.

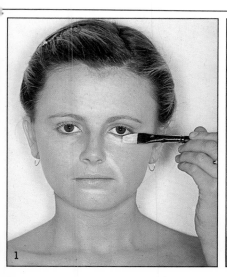

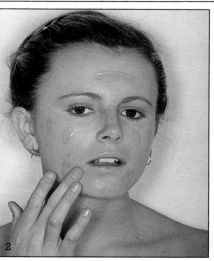

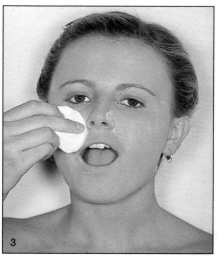

1. Start by covering shadows under the eyes by using a pale flesh colour cover cream stippled on lightly with a brush.

2. Foundation goes on next. Choose a shade that blends in with the colour of your neck, and apply it with smooth downward strokes.

3. Loose powder is used to set the make-up so that it lasts. Colourless translucent shades are best. Always apply with cotton wool.

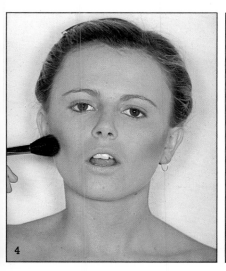

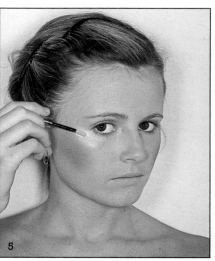

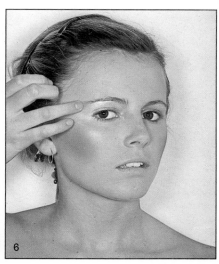

4. Using a big brush called a rouge mop, apply brown contour powder or a tawny blusher under the cheekbones to emphasize bone structure.

5. A shiny frosted highlighter in an ivory shade is used to highlight the top of the cheekbones, to give a subtle play of light and shade to the face.

6. To ensure that eye make-up lasts without going into little lines in the creases on the eye, use an ivory-toned water-based gloss over the lid.

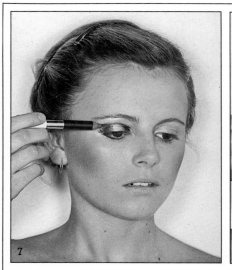

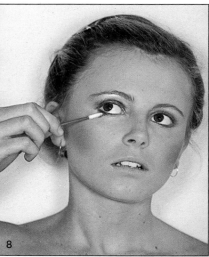

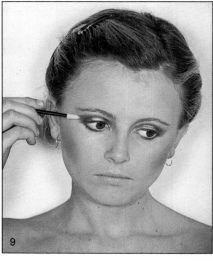

7 Apply a soft grey eye shadow crayon to contour the eye, shading it in above the crease.

8 To blend in eye shadow use a cotton bud on the lid and underneath the eye to give a soft natural looking effect.

9 Powder eye shadow is applied over the crayon to set the colour, using a little sponge applicator.

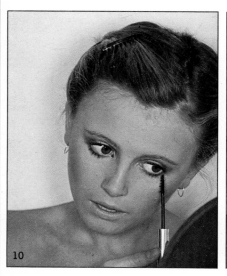

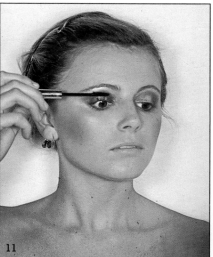

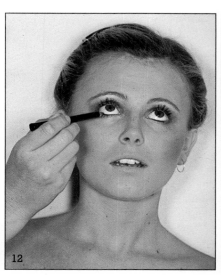

10 Apply mascara to bottom lashes first.

11 Then apply mascara to top lashes afterwards: this will help to prevent getting mascara on the brow bone.

12 Define the shape of the eye with a soft black kohl pencil applied inside the rim.

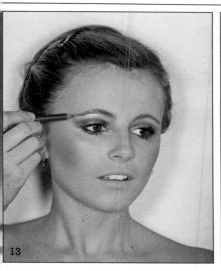
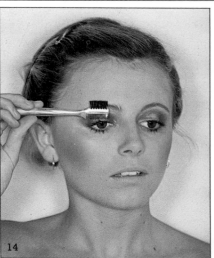
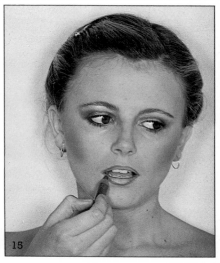

13

Pencilling eyebrows should always be done with little feathery strokes using a grey/brown coloured pencil.

14

After drawing in the eyebrows with pencil soften the line by using a little eyebrow brush.

15

To get a good contour to the lips draw in the outline with a pinky/brown lip pencil.

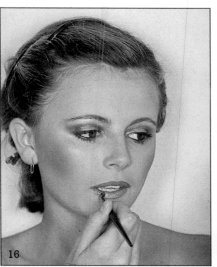
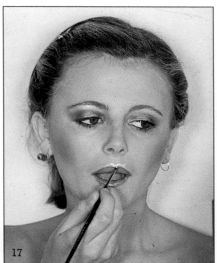
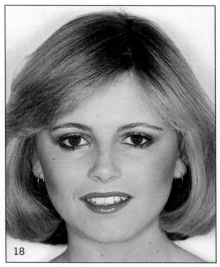

16

Apply lipstick with a brush, using a clear bright colour.

17

To emphasize the Cupid's bow of your lips, use the make-up artists' trick of putting pale flesh-tinted highlighter above the centre of the lips.

18

The final effect: hair brushed out, make-up finished; but despite all the care taken the look is natural and not artificial.

Shaders

Shaders come in cream stick or powder form: their colours are brown tones. I usually recommend the powder form because it is more stable and easier to apply. Because in the past so few people realized the purpose of shaders and knew how to use them, many of the best have now been discontinued by their manufacturers. But nearly all the leading contemporary make-up artists use shaders and I believe that the extra definition they give is important. Powder shaders are best applied with a big brush. Brushes are in fact an important part of the armoury you need to get the best out of your make-up.

Forget the traditional advice on using shaders, which was to suck your cheeks in and apply the shader down the hollows towards the mouth. The problem about doing this is that where the brush stops, you will get a brown blob by the side of your mouth. We always tell our clients that the way to put on shadow is to feel with their finger for the hollow below the line of their cheekbone. Load the brush with shader, use the hand to knock away any surplus colour, then stipple the shader on with the brush, working away from the mouth. It is important to keep the brush head pointing upwards, holding the brush near its head in the same way that you hold a pen. By pointing the brush upwards you will ensure that the shader goes on high enough, right under your cheekbones.

Blushers

Blushers are the modern version of rouge: like rouge, their purpose is to give a lively glow to the face. Blushers come in various colours; the most suitable are not always the ones which look the prettiest in the compact. For example, a tawny terracotta tone is usually much more flattering when on the face than a clear pink or coral. Blushers come in various forms: powder, gel, liquid and cream. I always recommend the powder form, because it is the most lasting and easiest to apply.

Blushers are applied to the face higher than shaders – on the top of the cheekbone. Be sure to keep the colour on the outside of the face, rather than towards the nose, since this is where your own natural colour is strongest. Blushers are best applied with a brush; you can use the same one as for your shader. Fill your brush, tap out the surplus with your hand, and then apply the blusher to the top of your cheekbones with a circular movement, clockwise and anti-clockwise. When your brush has emptied of blusher, take the brush up and down the side of your face towards the temples and down to your chin to distribute the residue of the colour evenly.

Highlighter

Highlighter is the last of the three facial contouring products – shader, blusher and highlighter. It goes above the cheekbone and above your blusher. Its purpose is to add a shine to the top of your cheekbones and to give a lively-looking gleam to your skin. Because the shine is so important, highlighters are always frosted and in pale ivory tones. They are normally in cream stick or powder form. Nearly every beauty manufacturer includes a highlighter in their range. As an alternative you can use any pale frosted eyeshadow powder or frosted eye crayon.

Cream stick and crayons are stroked on straight from the stick. To get the best effect with frosted powders you need to apply them with a piece of cotton wool, folded tightly, rolled into the powder and then applied to the top of the cheekbone and underneath the outer corner of the eye; turn the cotton wool over and buff up the shine. Highlighter completes the sculpturing of your face. We now move on to the eyes.

EYES

Eye make-up is important, because done well it can enhance the shape of your eyes – make small eyes look larger, pale eyes more definite, close-set eyes wider apart, deep-set eyes less deep set, and heavy-lidded eyes less lidded. A good eye make-up requires at least three shadows, because without these it is impossible to get sufficient play of light and shade to contour the eye. It is with contouring techniques that you effect the change of shape of your eye.

Eye make-up requires practice and you need to follow a basic technique. You prepare the canvas by applying a water-based eye gloss in a pale ivory shade over the whole eye area as a foundation for other shadows. This goes over the whole lid area from eyebrows down to the lashes. Use water-based glosses as these dry in contact with the warmth of the skin and do not melt and go into little lines in the folds of the eyelids, which used to happen with the old-fashioned soft cream shadows. The next colour you use can be in powder, crayon or cream form. What is important is that it should be in a dark contouring colour such as brown or grey. This colour goes above the crease of the eyelid. To put it on for the best effect, do not raise your eyebrow: look straight ahead into the mirror and feather the colour on in little strokes in an arc above the fold of the eye. Do not make the mistake of putting it in the crease. As I always say to clients, you do not talk to friends with your chin stuck up in the air; instead, pretend your mirror is the friend you are talking to and you will apply the colour as it is seen by other people.

The last colour you apply is a pale one, which should be keyed to what you are wearing: blue, green, lilac, mauve, olive or gold. This goes on the lid behind the lashes. These colours come in crayon, powder or cream form. If you know how to use them crayons are the most stable and easiest to blend. But it requires practice, plenty of cotton buds for blending, and a light touch in applying. Do not use crayons to draw lines as they will give you a harsh look, as well as dragging the delicate skin on the eyelids.

I find that many of my clients, who have a fair English colouring with sandy pale lashes, believe that they can only use pale eyeshadows. They usually add that they once experimented with brown or grey shadow, but looked as if they had been given a black eye. In fact anyone who has fair lashes and experiments with a darker than usual eyeshadow will give herself a fright if she makes up her eyes without mascara. If you are experimenting with eyeshadow colours, do put your mascara on first.

Mascara

Mascara is essential to any good eye make-up. In fact, I believe it to be the most important eye make-up accessory.

The purpose of mascara is not just to colour your lashes, but more important, to give an outline to the eyes of anyone with fair colouring. Even if you have dark eyelashes, you will still find that mascara helps emphasize the shape of the eye. Mascara on lashes acts as a natural eye shaper. If you are fair you must be generous in your use of it. It is not sufficient to give each eye a couple of timid dabs with the mascara brush, as the colour must go from the roots to the tips of the lashes to be effective.

I judge mascaras by their ability to remain smudge-proof: it is more important than water-proofing. Few of us spend our lives jumping in and out of swimming pools, whereas many of us suffer from smudging mascara, which gives us dark circles under our eyes. The reason for smudging, which is not generally understood, is that it is caused by mascara melting after contact with warm skin. Finding a smudge-proof mascara can be an extremely tedious and expensive pastime. You have to try a large number before you find one which is really stable. And you are not going to get much help from consultants in stores, selling only their own brand, or from chemists, who have not enough interest or experience.

I was asked recently to give my opinion on a mascara survey done by *Which?*. Much to my surprise I discovered that very few of my favourite and best-selling mascaras were included on their list. When I heard the nature of the test they had done to make their selection, I understood why this was so. *Which?* had put a whole lot of false lashes on to a sheet and applied a different mascara to each one. Water was then sprayed on to them. Any make of mascara which did not run was eligible to be included in their list. I pointed out that with my customers a smudge-proof mascara was more important than a water-proof one, and unless they could devise a test whereby they could mount lashes on warm moisturized skin and blink them frequently over a period to see which makes melted, there was no way that I felt their results were relevant to life.

Always put mascara on bottom lashes first, otherwise if you start with the top lashes and then open your eyes wide before the mascara dries, you will get little black smudges on the brow-bone.

Some women worry about mascara sticking the lashes together and making them look spiky. For this reason, directly after applying mascara, I always recommend using a clean brush to separate the lashes. A useful tip is that because the majority of photographers dislike lashes that look too heavily loaded with mascara, models often spend ten minutes after applying mascara separating their lashes with a hair pin to get a natural effect.

Never make up your eyes without having your emergency kit ready to rescue you should your mascara smudge or eyeshadow go on to your cheek instead of your eyelids. Dip one end of a cotton bud into non-oily eye make-up remover, and squeeze it out so that it is damp.

Eyeliner and Kohl Pencil
Although "out" according to fashion pundits, eyeliner is still a big seller in most beauty ranges. In my opinion the eyeliner look that dates you is a dark brown or black liner worn on its own, or with a pale shadow, or any eyeliner which is drawn in extended lines beyond the shape of the eye. Eyeliner in soft tones matching the current eyeshadow colours can be used effectively to enhance the shape of the eye without drawing attention to itself.

Today leading professional make-up artists use kohl pencils instead of eyeliner. The problem about kohl pencils is that they are difficult to use and you must know which brands are best. Only the very soft ones are easy to apply.

Kohl pencils should be applied inside the rim of the eye. Original kohl paste was black, but the modern pencils come in a variety of colours. Choose one which enhances the colour of your eyes or clothes.

EYEBROWS
You can do more to improve your looks by adjusting the shape of your eyebrows than by doing practically anything else. I know that if I am ever

doing a make-up demonstration, I always try to find a woman whose eyebrows are straggly and lack shape. A little tidying up can do wonders. Establishing a shape is best done by a professional. It is not particularly expensive and is money well spent.

After your eyebrows have been shaped, you usually need to add definition. The way you do this has changed a lot in the last fifteen years. It is more important to define the shape of the eye with shadows and highlighters than to draw attention to eyebrows with heavy pencilling. In fact since women learnt to define eye shape by using eyeliner, emphasizing eyebrows has become less important. Current eyebrow shaping tends to follow the natural shape: pin-thin lines are out, and so is the trick of having a thick beginning tapering off to a thin line. The best way of defining your eyebrows is with a soft grey brown pencil, applied in light feathery strokes: brush the pencilling with an eyebrow brush, following the natural line.

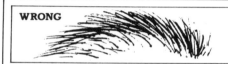

WRONG

Brows that aren't properly shaped can look heavy and untidy: straggling hairs spoil the shape and get in the way of eye make-up.

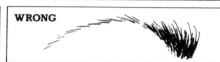

WRONG

Brows shouldn't be plucked into pin-thin arcs with heavy clumps at the ends that look like commas on either side of the bridge of the nose.

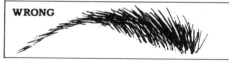

WRONG

Brows that are too heavy near the nose and too thin at the ends tend to look vampishly arched like a '50s screen siren.

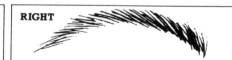

RIGHT

Brows should be shaped into a light-looking arc that has a gradual sweep so that they enhance the eyes.

LIPSTICK

More women complain about the difficulties of buying lipstick than any other cosmetic. First, finding the right colour is more difficult than one thinks, and most customers complain that they have to buy half a dozen before they get one they really like. Certainly, from my own experience, once I have found a colour, I stick to it and wear it with everything. The concept that you should have a variety of lip colours to compliment everything you wear is a nice idea but it is only really applicable when you are young.

The other big problem is how to prevent lipstick coming off on cups and glasses. All my customers over thirty-five complain bitterly that lipsticks have become less and less stable over the years. They remember the dryer texture of a more indelible type of lipstick which contained more eosin, the pigment colour that gives tone to lipstick and makes it last. With these more lasting lipsticks you were encouraged to apply them and then blot on a tissue so that you got a matt, non-smear finish. This became the hallmark of the older woman, and as a result young women stopped wearing lipstick altogether, preferring to cover their lips with pan-stick. Today colour is back in lipstick, but unfortunately present fashion is not likely to produce a lasting, non-smearing, shiny, see-through lipstick. But there are a number of things you can do to make your lipstick stay on better.

1 Use a crayon as an outline because they are more stable than lipstick, and they give a good lasting contour to the lips. Crayons you use on your lips must be in pigment tones such as freckle or bruise colours. A freckle brown crayon makes a perfect outline for any of your golden red lipsticks. Bruise brown crayons are the mauve brown colours which are very close to the natural colour of your lips but darker, and these make an ideal outline for all pink and blue-red lipstick colours. These pigment crayons are much more successful outliners than bright pink or scarlet lipstick crayons.

2 Take a tip from the professionals and apply your lipstick with a brush. The first application of the day should be done in this way because the colour goes on thinly and evenly and you will find that the result will be more lasting. Personally I find that I need to touch up during the day, and for this I use the lipstick in the normal way.

3 Add shine afterwards with a touch of transparent or, better still, frosted transparent lip gloss. The advantage of frosted lip glosses is that by being light reflecting they have a softening effect on too bright colours. If you prefer to blot your lipstick – and this sometimes seems to help make it last better – do so, but put a touch of lip gloss on afterwards – then at least the cup smear is likely to be that of more gloss than colour.

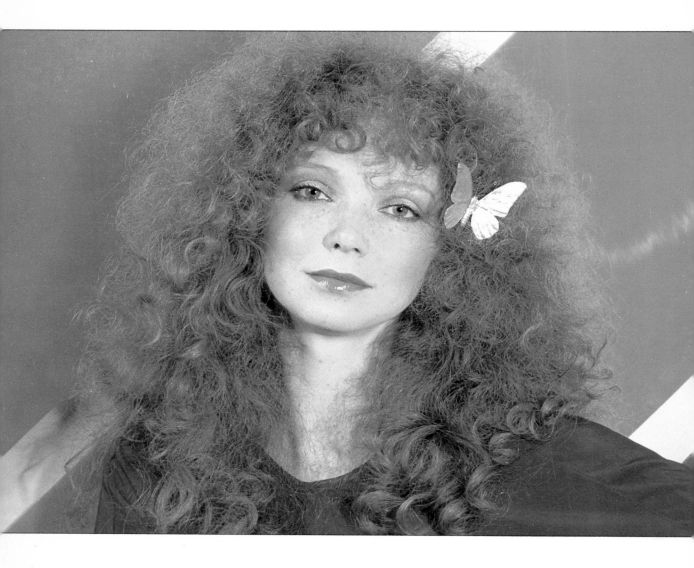

Make-up for a redhead calls for a soft golden skin tone that will give warmth to the complexion and plenty of emphasis on the eyes in order to give them definition and get rid of that sandy albino look.

The foundation used here is Princess Galitzine's Velvet Matte 01, set with Max Factor's Purified Finishing Powder shade Transparent Matte.

Cheeks are contoured with Elizabeth Arden's Venetian Glow blusher, and highlighted with Helena Rubinstein's Silvergold Frost.

Charles of the Ritz Roseshine is used on eyelids with Elizabeth Arden's Golden Grape eye-shadow. Princess Galitzine's Sapphire Blue kohl pencil is used inside the eye and Lancôme's black mascara on the lashes. Her lipstick is Elizabeth Arden's Bronze Lamé, with Elizabeth Arden's gloss over the top.

Butterfly ornament by Adrien Mann and make-up by Melanie of the Face Place.

COLOUR SENSE

Colour plays a critical part today in any good make-up and those lucky enough to be born with a good colour sense will find themselves with a great advantage. In fact as the selection of colours in make-up ranges grows every year, so does the importance of having colour sense.

Up to a few years ago it was possible to make up to basic rules, and your choice of colour was not critical. But the dramatic change in eye make-up and the increasingly sophisticated selection of colours in complexion tones have completely altered the situation.

Even ten years ago eye make-up was straightforward and simple. It was matched to the colour of your eyes. Blue-eyed blondes used blue eye-shadows while brown-eyed brunettes used green or brown shadows. Today, with the changing emphasis on the face, eye colour is influenced not only by what you are wearing, but also by whether it is for day or evening.

So how do you set about deciding on the colours that will make you look your best?

To start at the beginning, forget all the preconceived ideas about choosing a foundation colour. Blondes certainly do not look their best in pink-toned make-up, which they frequently imagine matches their "milk and roses" skin. Because they often have a strong colouring of pink in their skin, a flat beige tone will normally give them a more natural-looking and attractive effect.

Women with sallow skins need to use a foundation which will liven up their skin tone, but be careful about choosing a colour with too much pink or peach. Apart from the fact that peach tones react to the oil in the skin after you have worn them for a while and go orangey, there is too much yellow in a peach tone to make it a satisfactory colour choice for someone with a sallow skin. If you have a very sallow skin the best corrective tone is a mauvey pink, and this is really best used as an undercoat in the form of a tinted moisturizer, covered with a beige foundation.

Another problem for brunettes is that they often have very pale skins which can look lifeless with dark brown hair. Their make-up needs to add warmth to the skin so that there is less contrast in tone, but a foundation with too much pink or peach will not be as appropriate as a golden beige tone.

I continually find that most women have a very strong antipathy to

Actress Lalla Ward has a good natural colour sense. Sarah at the Face Place created a make-up that would be complementary to her blond looks and her scarlet tunic.

Lalla needs a golden beige shade of make-up to warm her fair complexion. To give emphasis to the eyes Sarah used gold bronze and russet tones carefully blended together, yet positive enough to balance the strong lipstick colour which was chosen to match the scarlet tunic. This colour is called Wildfire in Mary Quant's Soft Machine lip pencil range, and in order to give plenty of gloss to the lips, which prevents a bright colour like this one from looking too hard, Sarah put a colourless Mary Quant lip gloss called Glosspot over the top.

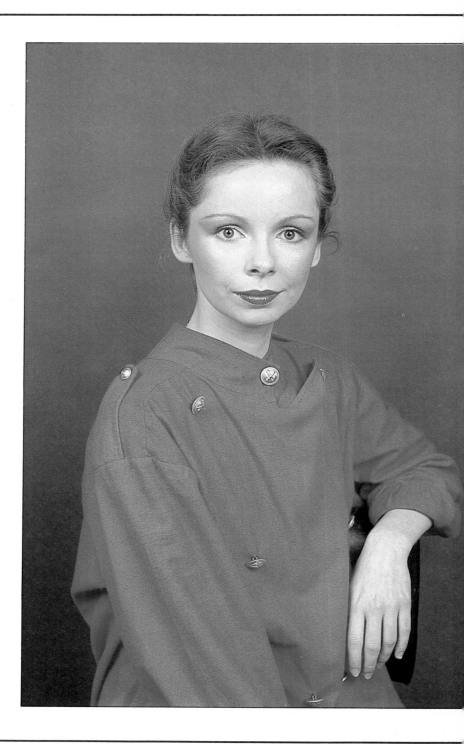

beige make-up tones. There are probably two reasons for this. First, a beige tone does not look appealing in the bottle and certainly needs to be tried on the face to get any idea of its effect. The other reason is that because it tones down redness, rosy-faced women feel that it makes them look ill; in fact, as your redness is never in the right place, it is best added with a blusher.

The importance of beige-tone foundations is that they make the perfect basic skin tone for rouge and blusher which should always be used to give a glow to the face.

When choosing a rouge or blusher, forget the old idea that it should tone in with your lipstick. The cleverness about modern rouge, particularly blusher tones, is that it is formulated to blend with foundation colours. It is difficult to find the best rouge colours without trying them on the face, because in the packs tawny colours look so unappealing. It is only when they are on your face that you realize how effective they are. The blusher colours to be avoided are the ones that look brightest in the compact, so do not be beguiled into choosing pinks and clear corals. Instead you will find that the unlikely looking browny-brick tone will give you a much more natural looking glow.

One of the factors which people often underestimate in their skin is the melanin or pigment. As you get older, the melanin remains nearer the surface and affects the way your make-up colours look on your skin. However fair she is, any woman over forty-five will always have much too much melanin content in her skin to be able to wear a pale pink or pale peach make-up. That clear pink tone foundation which looked so good on your skin when you were in your early twenties will look very made-up if you continue to wear it as you get older, whereas a light tan shade will blend in and look completely natural.

The other important factor to remember when choosing make-up colours is the effect of light on the skin. Although daylight can be much colder than electric light, it does not distort colour in the same way as artificial lighting which drains colour and flattens your features. This means that on the whole you need to wear stronger colours at night. For instance, because it is a primary colour, blue eye make-up worn during the day will often tend to give a more made-up look to the eyes than, say, a natural pigment tone brown. Yet a brown eye make-up for evening will lack the impact of blue, green or purple shadows. At night it is also important to wear a stronger brown face-shaper and a warmer rouge to give more emphasis to your features.

An important point to remember about make-up today is that eyes and lips should balance. Wearing too strong a lipstick and virtually no eye

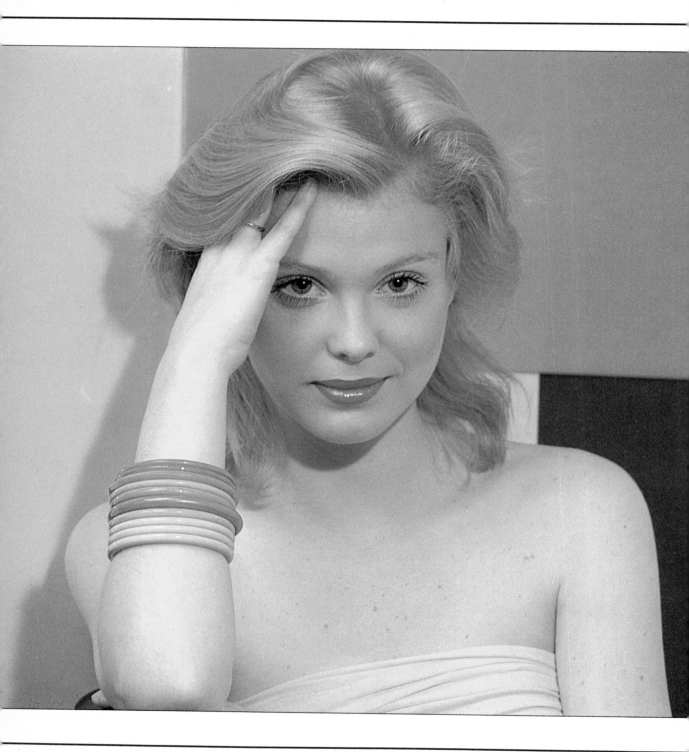

make-up, or – just as bad – heavily outlined eyes and a pale mouth, gives an unbalanced look to the face.

An important development in recent years has been the introduction of pearlized or frosted colours. These are now mainly used for eye colours. Their purpose is to add light and shade to the area above the eye. The principle on which they work is that the frosted colour brings into prominence features such as the brow-bone which you wish to highlight.

Pearlized colours work best when teamed with the more solid matt-looking colours, and in fact most eye-kits today combine pearlized and matt colours. While pearlized colours highlight the areas on which they are used, matt colours are used for emphasizing shaded areas such as the crease of the eye.

Because I find that so many women ask me for some basic rules on how to start using colours to suit their skin and hair tones, I have included a chart on pages 122 and 123. Any guide such as this will tend to oversimplify and it will be of very limited use to those who have a developed colour sense and have spent time in experimenting with make-up colours. But if you are one of those who does not know where to begin, I think you will find it of some value; and once you have gained the initial confidence, you will be surprised how quickly you are able to develop your own colour sense. As in so many other aspects of beauty, it is the first steps which are always the hardest. I hope that the chart will help you over these first steps, which I find inhibit so many women.

You will notice on the chart that certain colours are constant, regardless of fashion. Foundation and blusher are always based on your colouring, whereas eyes and lips can pick up colour from what you are wearing. You will also notice that in general recommended colours for evening are warmer than those for day, to counteract the flattening effect of artificial lighting.

Remember that regardless of your age, you cannot use all the colours in the spectrum. You are limited by your basic colouring. I often find that a fair woman will bring in a colour picture from a fashion magazine of a model or film star such as Sophia Loren, and ask us to create the same look for her. Such an experiment is always a failure, because you must keep to the general rules of colour coordination.

One of the main difficulties in choosing colour is buying cosmetics in the artificial light of department stores. Many manufacturers are unfortunately aware that their products will be seen for the first time in this artificial light and they tend to doctor foundations and powders with pink or peach pigments, so that they look acceptable in store lighting. This often means that once you get into the daylight you find you have chosen too hot a colour.

Day-time make-up for blondes should be relatively simple: to be well done it relies on several well-chosen products such as foundation, loose powder, blusher, eyeshadows, mascara and lipstick.

The girl in this picture has a golden-toned make-up in contrast to the fairness of her blond hair. She is wearing Elizabeth Arden's Toasty Beige Flawless Finish foundation; Max Factor's colourless Swedish Formula Transculent Matte powder; Mary Quant's Toffee Blush Baby blusher; Charles of the Ritz's Softshine Eye Shadow Pommade with Almay's Woodtones Powder Shadow eyeshadows; Mary Quant's Lashtint mascara; and Leichner's Close-to-Tawny lipstick.

To achieve the most effective contemporary look, blondes should forget the old rules about choosing peach or pink foundations and blue or green shadows to match the colour of their eyes. They will find that the monotone effect achieved with tawny colours gives a more natural, sculptured look to the face.

BLONDES/REDHEADS

OUTFIT COLOUR	Blue Green	Yellow Brown	Lilac Purple Red	Black White
EYESHADOW COLOUR **DAY**	Grey/Blue Ivory/Green	Ivory/Brown	Ivory/Grey Tourmaline	Grey Brown Ivory
EVENING	Grey/Pink Grape Gold/Brown Olive	Cinnamon Brown/Gold	Pink Grape Purple	Yellow Green Grape Pink Blue Gold
FOUNDATION COLOUR **DAY**	Beige	Beige	Beige	Beige
EVENING	Gold beige	Gold beige	Gold beige	Gold beige
BLUSHER COLOUR **DAY**	Frosted Peach	Frosted Peach	Frosted Peach	Frosted Peach
EVENING	Terracotta	Terracotta	Terracotta	Terracotta
LIPSTICK COLOUR **DAY**	Pink	Gold Bronze	Grape	Plum Scarlet
EVENING	Plum	Brown Red	Petunia	Burgundy Scarlet
NAILS COLOUR	Pink tone	Bronze tone	Pink tone	Pink Bronze tones

BRUNETTES & DARKER/GREYHEADS

Blue Green	Yellow Brown	Lilac Purple Red	Black White	OUTFIT COLOUR
Brown/Turquoise Ivory Brown Olive	Ivory/ Cinnamon Brown	Pink Grey Grape	Ivory Rust Grey	EYESHADOW COLOUR DAY
Brown/Gold Pink mauve Aubergine	Yellow rust Gold Rust Brown	Burgundy Blue Ivory Pink	Cinnamon Turquoise	EVENING
Honey/ gold	Honey/ gold	Honey/ gold	Honey/ gold	FOUNDATION COLOUR DAY
Tan gold	Tan gold	Tan gold	Tan gold	EVENING
Frosted Rose	Frosted Rose	Frosted Rose	Frosted Rose	BLUSHER COLOUR DAY
Copper Rose Tawny Wine	Copper Rose	Copper Rose Tawny Wine	Copper Rose	EVENING
Gold Coral Pink	Copper Coral Red	Gold Pink	Copper Coral Red	LIPSTICK COLOUR DAY
Coral Red	Brown Coral Red Red	Burgundy Red	Brown Red	EVENING
Coral tone	Copper tone	Plum	Copper tone Coral	NAILS COLOUR

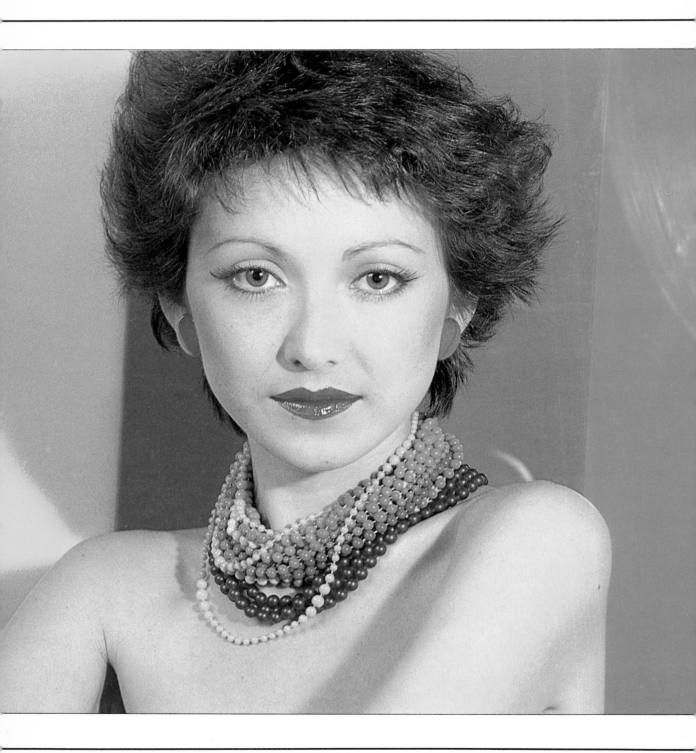

Women often ask me about the extent to which they ought to change their make-up to match what they are wearing. Frequently this thought has been stimulated by a fashion promotion for new colours in a magazine such as *Vogue*. The value of such a promotion for make-up is that it creates interest in new colours and encourages women to experiment.

Most make-up artists advocate adjusting your make-up to what you are wearing and, as shown on the chart, altering your eye and lip make-up colours to pick up your fashion colours. While I believe that this can be very effective on a young face, I find that your scope becomes more limited as you get older. In general, once over forty, while it is possible to use blue, green and mauve colours, the more you keep to your natural skin tones such as basic brown and grey, the less likely you are to appear over made-up.

Make-up colours cannot be dealt with in isolation without discussing clothes, because to get the best out of both they should complement each other.

I think it is important to make it clear that there are very few hard and fast rules and that nothing can improve on a good colour instinct. But having said that, there are a few basic guidelines that can sometimes help and which are worth bearing in mind.

1 White, off-white and cream are probably the most flattering fashion colours for everyone.

2 Sallow-skinned people should avoid all colours with a yellow base such as sage green, khaki, gold, beige and muddy brown.

3 If you have florid cheeks avoid blue-pink tones such as cyclamen, mauve, purple or magenta, worn close to the face.

4 Natural blondes and women with grey hair will sometimes find that a lot of bright colours will tend to make them look washed out. Restrict them to a bright accessory such as a scarf or blouse. Being fair myself, I find that black, navy and drab colours are more flattering for me.

5 Tanned skins look best with white or clear bright colours rather than black, which can look hot.

Brunette Vivienne Lynn's make-up is her own creation: she took as her inspiration the pale look of Kabuki, the traditional Japanese theatre make-up, and wears her own version of it for parties. To achieve it she uses Almay's Soft Moon Beige foundation with Japanese rice powder over the top, and she puts a bright pink rouge high on her cheekbones. For her eyes she blends three or four colours from the Cosmetics à la Carte Colour Box, putting yellow, ochre, and gold shadows together and wears false eyelashes, Eylure's Naturalites I, to give more definition to her eyes. Her lipstick is a bright clear red from the Leichner Theatrical lipstick palette.

Vivienne knows exactly what to use to achieve the right colour values: a pale foundation makes lipstick and rouge look stronger; and when she wants a more natural look she wears a darker, golden-tanned foundation so that her lipstick and eye make-up look softer.

Vivienne's hair is by John Freida, jewellery by Adrien Mann.

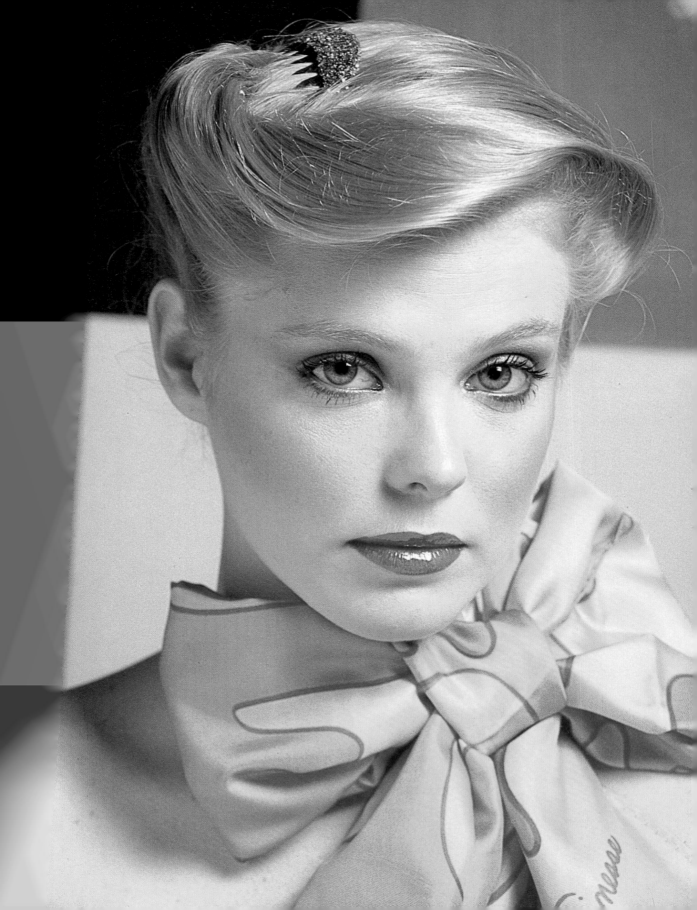

Of course there are women with a highly developed colour sense who break all the rules all the time and yet always look good. But unless you have their confidence and flair, which cannot be taught, you will be safer to bear some of these guidelines in mind when choosing clothes.

For an authoritative last word I went to one of the foremost fashion leaders in this country, Lady Rendlesham, who runs the Saint Laurent Rive Gauche and Chloe shops. She stressed the point that one is always restricted in one's choice of colour by the fashion colours of the moment and that if it is a fashionable look you wish to achieve, it is vital to start with the colours that are in at the time of your choice. In general, she feels that bright colours look best on dark-haired women but blues in every shade and tone are always good on blondes.

BLACK IS BEAUTIFUL

This is a slogan which can certainly be applied to many coloured girls today. But they are outnumbered by the many others who find it difficult to adapt standard cosmetic ranges to their dark skins. Unfortunately, although there have been several attempts to market a special range for dark skins in this country, most of these have failed. Women with dark skins, whether Asian or West Indian, do have to find colours in the existing Northern European ranges which are suitable for them. But there really is no need to be despondent and to give up trying. It is the girls who have taken time and trouble to find their way around the colours that are available who are generally the ones who look so good. I have spoken to many of them, including pop star celebrities and business girls, and from the tips they have given me I have compiled some basic rules.

Foundation

The first requirement for a dark skin is a good foundation that will enhance the colour in a subtle way and still look natural. As one West Indian girl said to me recently, "When I look closely at my skin, I see that it is purple, plum and pink as well as brown, and I need a basic colour which will play down these variations in tone, and give me a smooth, even finish."

The best sort of colour for a dark skin is a transparent bronzing gel. These look like Marmite when they come out of the tube, but smooth on evenly to give a slightly warmer deep-tan glow to the skin. Otherwise the best colours for this type of skin are produced by theatrical ranges such as Max Factor and Leichner, and have colour names such as blend of brown, blend of tawny, blend of copper, and café bronze.

Evening make-up should be stronger and more dramatic and so will involve more products. The main reason for this is that artificial lighting has the effect of draining colour from your face and of flattening your features.

Though more stylized than the day-time look, this make-up retains the same colour tones as a contrast to the blond hair. The foundation is Germaine Monteil's Superglow Ivory Beige with Geminesse Translucent Finishing Powder; the cheek shader is by Biba with Mary Quant's Paprika Blush Baby and Miss Selfridge's No. 3 highlighter on the top of the cheekbones. On the eyes the shading is achieved with Charles of the Ritz's Softshine and Seagreen Mist, Miss Selfridge's Gold No. 1 and Fabergé's Babe Roast Chestnut shadows. Galitzine Black and Silvery Blue kohl pencils outline the eye. The lipstick is Charles of the Ritz's Papete with plenty of shine, and Natural Gloss by Leichner.

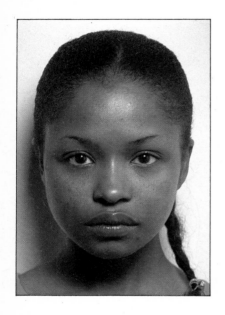

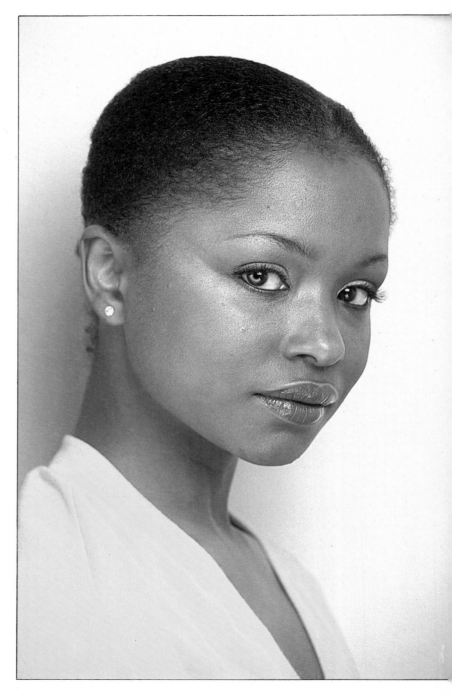

Girls with dark skins will have
less choice of make-up products
available to them. Yet these two
pictures show that make-up
skills can produce as great a
transformation to girls with
dark skins as to anyone else.

The make-up in the
photograph on the right was by
Sarah at the Face Place. She used
Leichner's Blend of Brown
foundation with Revlon's Honey
Brown Frost to shade the
cheekbones, and Biba's
Ladybird blusher and Innoxa's
Truly Peach highlighter.
Eyeshadow colours were
Golden Sun by Galitzine, with
Mary Quant's Shades of Plum
and Miss Selfridge's shiny No. 13
and No. 1. Eyes were outlined
with Galitzine's black kohl
pencil. The lipstick was Yves
St Laurent's No. 13 with
Elizabeth Arden's Gloss Over
lip gloss.

For a coffee-coloured skin most standard European ranges include a warm coppery tan shade, and this, or the fake tanning gels, is suitable for livening up your colour. Avoid sandy yellow tones which will make your skin look sallower.

Rouges

Most of the currently popular rosy pink shades of rouge look very attractive on a dark skin. Cream or gel rouges usually look the most effective, but are not as lasting as powder rouges. Although the maximum colour should be applied to the cheekbones, it is important to take the colour around the outside of the face in order to give a more all-over glow.

Eye Make-up

Most dark-skinned girls emphasize the importance of using natural-looking amber brown and grey eyeshadow colours, rather than garish blues and greens teamed with white highlighters that can look hard and chalky. Many also rely on black kohl pencils used inside the rim of the eye to give definition. As one of them said to me recently, "I think Eastern women knew what they were doing when they discovered kohl – it does wonders for people with a dark colouring."

One of the most successful eyeshadow colours for a dark skin is a pinky brown which teams well with garnet, plum and ambered rose colours on the lids. Frosted highlighters in an ivory/peach tone are effective for giving a soft play of light and shade to the eye area.

For girls with very dark skins, dark brown, black or grey cake eyeliner applied with water can be used as shadow to give depth to the socket of the eye.

Lipsticks

Transparent bronze, copper and burgundy tones look best on dark lips: bright scarlet reds and pinks usually look too hard. Wear your colour with plenty of transparent lip gloss over the top.

In the evening, because of the yellow tones in electric lighting, you can afford to introduce more red into your lip colour. Give your lips more definition by using a deep ruby or brown/red lipstick that can look very good after dark.

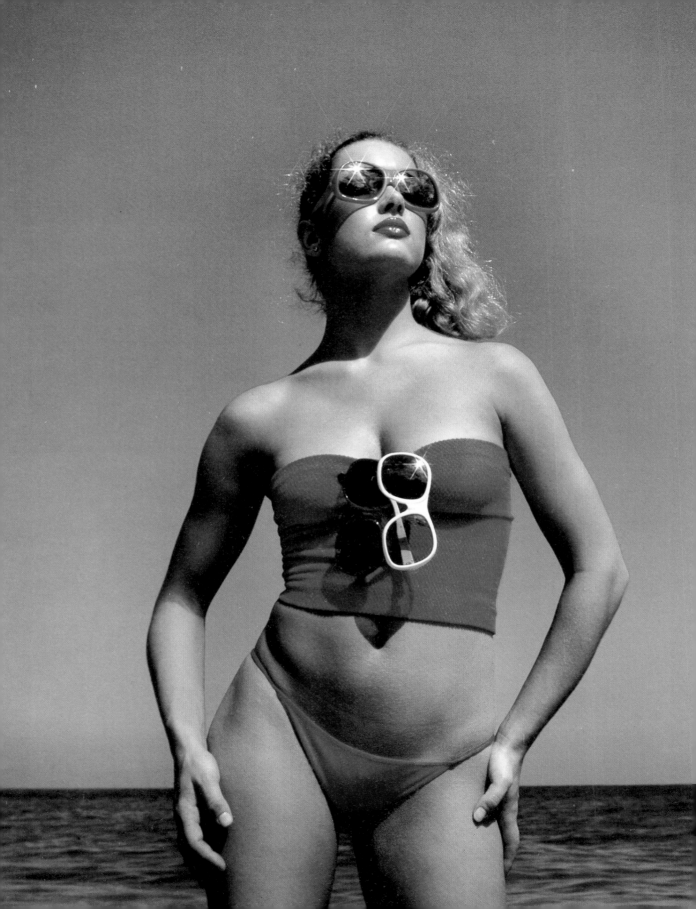

SUN-LOOKS

Although many early civilizations worshipped the sun, the idea of using the sun to give you a suntanned look is very recent. Most of us find it surprising that right up to 1914 people went to the South of France to get away from our northern winters. The idea of going there in the summer did not occur to them, as the sun at that time of the year would have seemed to be too hot and uncomfortable.

It was Coco Chanel, the setter of so many fashion trends, who pioneered the suntanned look. She had the type of skin which tanned and looked at its best when brown. With all the changes in style and attitude of the twenties, this new brown look quickly became popular; in particular, it was seen as the prerogative of the leisured classes who could afford holidays in the sun.

Today, a tan is considered not only attractive in itself, but to make a person seem healthy, sexually provocative, fit, relaxed, prestigious and fashionable.

Quite apart from subjective judgements which people make about each other and which are affected by how we look, a darkened skin does produce certain physical changes, such as producing a bright, white-eyed look, which we associate with general healthiness: this sets up a further contrast between the whites of the eyes and the pupils, so that the pupils and irises look darker and larger. In short we look livelier and healthier.

It is not surprising that the sun has created a whole new industry in itself. Quite apart from the proliferation of sun preparations such as protective creams, fake tans, sun blocks and after tans, items such as sun lamps, solaria, beach clothes and sunglasses are all big business in themselves. In fact, sunglasses have not only become a major fashion accessory in their own right, but they have greatly influenced the design of ordinary spectacles towards better-looking frames and larger lenses. Most of the leading fashion designers from Saint Laurent to Mary Quant have designed their own ranges of sunglasses; so successful have they been that the old adage no longer applies about "men not making passes at girls who wear glasses". Indeed,

---

Looking your best in the sun is a more complicated process than many women realize. Plenty of thought has to be given to sun specs and bikinis, and it is essential to prepare your skin carefully beforehand and to use suncreams as protection.

131

some girls feel naked without their "sun specs", wearing them throughout the winter in softer tints.

Although the sun may make you look great, it is important to realize that the sun and sunbathing are not going to do you or your skin any good in the long run. A growing number of dermatologists and beauty experts are agreed that the sun will age your skin more quickly than anything else.

This is very much borne out by the fact that many Australian women who spend a large part of their life in the sun have skins which become heavily lined and unevenly pigmented in later life. It is probably more than a coincidence that some specialists believe that the incidence of skin cancer amongst Europeans who live in warm climates, such as Australia and Florida, is higher than elsewhere in the world. Nor should we forget that the Arabs who have for centuries lived under the burning sun have kept their faces and bodies covered. Years of living under the boiling sun have in fact taught them the most practical way of coping with it.

The unwelcome truth is that the only people whom the sun benefits are those with young greasy skins, as it helps to dry up their spots and certainly has a short-term beneficial effect; paradoxically, hot climates have a devastatingly bad effect on people with cystic acne (lumpy blind spots which never come to a head).

Sunbathing and the tanned look are now so much part of our life and fashion that it is quite pointless to tell you not to sunbathe, and of course nothing can look more glamorous or attractive than a beautifully tanned face and body. But at least be careful and follow a few basic rules.

Men often ask me why we need to take so much trouble when we sunbathe. After all, "God made us as we are, and didn't mean us to add those modern products to our skin." The problem is that we do not exactly lead the lives that man was born to live. In the days of primitive man, the skin colour of a normally pigmented person living in a temperate zone changed according to the season. Man was far more adaptable than he is today. Today we tend to control our own climate, as we adjust it in our homes, offices and factories through central heating, by the clothes we wear and the environment in which we live. We adapt our surroundings to our requirements instead of the other way round.

In effect, a white man living in a temperate climate has to be far more careful when he goes out of his normal environment in exposing his skin to ultra-violet light, than does a black man living in a tropical climate. But when a black man comes to live in a temperate zone, his skin, over a period of time, loses some of its melanin content, and when he returns to his tropical environment, he has to be careful when first exposed again to ultra-violet rays.

The real danger period for burning is before you have turned brown and before the melanin or pigment in your skin has had time to come up to the surface as protection. The idea that exposing your skin to the sun works on the same principle as placing toast under a grill is a fallacy. Tanning results from a process inside the skin brought about by the action of the sun's ultra-violet rays. When you sunbathe, these rays stimulate the lower skin cells into producing more pigment or melanin, which comes to the surface as protection against burning. This is a slow process that varies with every type of skin: it can be at least two days before the tanned pigment is evenly distributed and if yours is a fair, dry skin it will take even longer. This explains the apparently unjust disparity between a dark, oily skin and the fair skin of, say, a redhead, who finds a painful crimson burn almost impossible to avoid.

The real key is to take sunbathing very slowly in the first three or four days of your holiday. Let me give you an important warning about one of the effects of sunburn few women are aware of. If you have a fair complexion, sunburn can break the tiny capillaries just under the surface of your skin and cause blotchy redness. Once this has happened, there is literally nothing you can do, except use make-up to hide the red patches on your cheeks which will stay with you for life. Unfortunately this is an effect which few women take seriously until it happens. It is a problem I am particularly aware of, because every year women come to me with broken veins and ask what I can do to help them: the only answer I have is to cover them with make-up. For skiers with fair skins, the risk can be even greater; the reflected sun on snow is twice as burning and red-apple cheeks can be a legacy for life.

A dermatologist to whom I send a number of my clients warns that in his experience a lot of unnecessary sun damage can also be done to children by lack of care at home. Mothers often think nothing of leaving children out of doors in a pram to roast on a sunny day without giving them any protection; there are a number of people with sun-reddened skins, who are paying the price of this type of neglect when young.

Having warned you of the dangers of the sun, let me now tell you what you can do to ensure that you get the benefit of a good suntan. As I have said earlier in this book, the best looks need time and trouble to achieve – they seldom happen automatically. Suntanning is no exception; a good suntan starts well before you go into the sun.

BEFORE YOU GO

The best way to prepare your skin for the sun is with a sun lamp, because it will bring the melanin up to the surface of your skin. I am not very enthusiastic about home sun lamps: although they are strong enough to damage your skin if used carelessly, they are not sufficiently powerful to give you any colour, and the limited spread of the ultra-violet rays means that you have to keep moving yourself or the lamp to get an even treatment. Unless you are very experienced in the use of sun lamps, I would strongly urge you to go to a good salon.

Beauty salons have many advantages when it comes to getting a tan from a sun lamp. The art of preparing for a good tan is more involved than first meets the eye, and most beauticians are very experienced in advising you on how your skin will react, about exposure times, if and when to use protective creams and goggles, and what kind of protection you should have for your hair.

They also use more powerful lamps, which need to be strictly supervised (in London, for instance, the operator has to be approved by the local council). As the manufacturers introduce new lamps, they are becoming more sophisticated all the time. Some of the newest and most effective come from Germany, and are beginning to revolutionize the sun-lamp market. They incorporate a number of radiation tubes which simulate the non-burning long wave UVA rays of the sun. These new UVA lamps are a great improvement on the old-style quartz and mercury vapour lamps because they colour the skin – you do go brown – and because they filter off the burning short-wave UVB and UVC rays, there is no risk of redness or peeling. It is also possible to use them with much longer exposure times so that results are obtained considerably more quickly. The majority of these lamps are designed as sunbeds and brown you back and front at the same time – you don't have to turn over, as was necessary with the old-style lamps. Because the tubes do not burn you on contact with them, the lamps are also much easier and safer to use.

These new lamps are unfortunately more expensive than previous lamps: they can cost up to £3000 to buy, so it is only the successful salons that can afford the latest models and only a very few people can afford to have them at home.

In a beauty salon, you will normally find that you need a course of treatments and, except for the very latest and most modern UVA machines we have discussed, sun lamps will not give you very much colour: what they

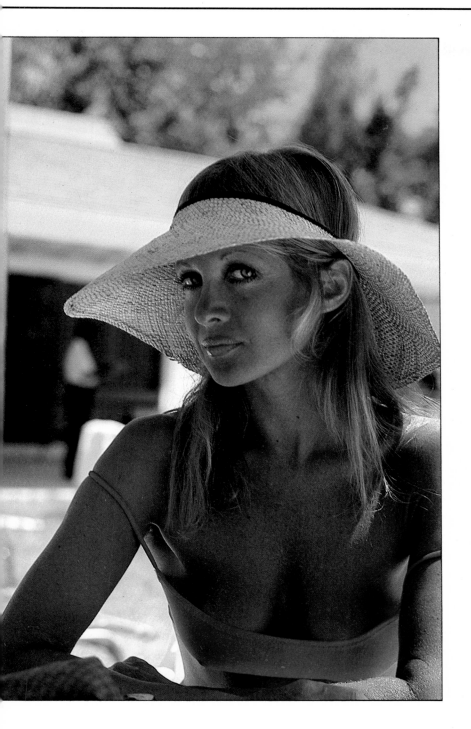

If you have a fair northern skin that does not really like the sun and will not tan easily, it is only sensible to give your face as much protection as you can. This is particularly so during the first few days you are on holiday in the sun. A wide-brimmed sun hat is a must for many women especially in the middle of the day when the sun's rays are at their most burning. If you are going to sit in the sun for a long time, you should also cover your hair, otherwise the sun can make it dry and brittle; and if you use bleaches or colourants on your hair, be careful or the colour can be badly affected.

One of the greatest
changes in beauty
treatments in recent
years has been the
invention of the new
UVA sun lamps.
Developed in Germany,
they have achieved the
objective which
everyone has been
hankering after for many
years. They give colour
to the skin without
burning, because they
filter out the burning
UVB and UVC rays of
the sun.

There are various
types of lamp. The one
in this picture is an
upright cabinet in which
you stand and get an
all-round tan. Unlike the
old lamps, you can have
twenty to thirty minutes'
exposure from the very
first day.

Alternative models of
UVA lamps vary from
couches which you lie
on, to a head and
shoulders lamp. These
lamps have been
available only for the
last eighteen months,
but can be found in
salons throughout the
country.

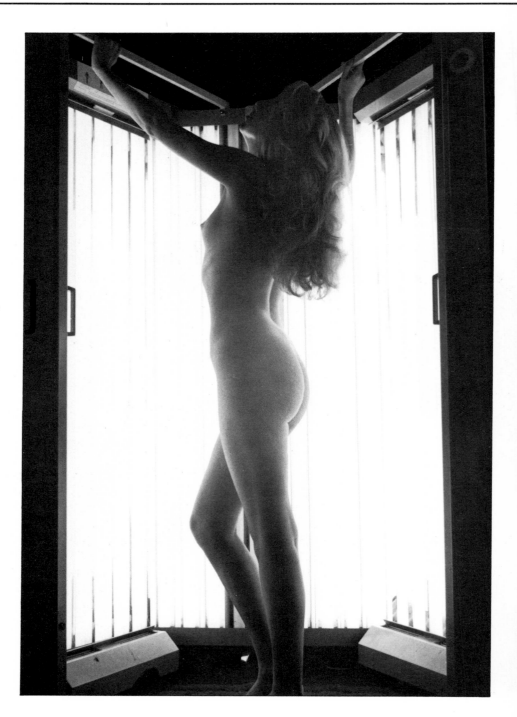

will do is to prepare your skin so that it does not burn easily when you first sit in the sun, and will brown quickly and evenly.

If you wish to look brown immediately on arrival in the sun, I recommend using an artificial overnight tan. These products are not just superficial skin colourants; they actually cause a chemical reaction in the skin four to five hours after application, when a pigment called melanoid appears in your skin which resembles the brown melanin pigment produced by the sun's ultra-violet rays. Because the colour comes from inside the skin having been activated by the product, it will not wash off and only fades gradually. The modern versions have improved enormously on the early prototype lotions of ten years ago when it was impossible to see which areas you had covered and which you had missed; the newest lotions have a smooth creamy consistency, so are applied easily and give an even coverage. To prevent staining it is sensible either to wear rubber gloves or to wash your hands immediately after applying the lotion. Before applying use plenty of moisturizing cream, particularly on rough areas like elbows, heels and knees so that the colour does not collect in these areas.

These products can be used either on your face or body. If you have never applied them before to your body, I recommend going to a salon which specializes in fake-take application as you need to be quite experienced to get an even tan all over without your skin looking streaked and patchy. They are particularly effective on your face and give you a convincing golden tan, and they are easy to apply to the face and go on smoothly. You will need two to three applications, one per day, to build up the colour. You can, of course, wear a fake tan any time during the year and it will always give you a healthy-looking appearance.

There is another type of fake tan, which is purely a temporary skin colourant, and which can be washed off at will. As there is no point in applying this before you go on holiday it will be discussed later in this chapter in the section dealing with make-up.

One of the least attractive aspects of a holiday in the sun is to come out of the water either with no mascara or with it running down your face. If you are fair, try getting your eyelashes tinted before going away. I am always surprised how few women are aware of this simple treatment and of the difference it can make. It gives the same effect as wearing mascara, but it has the advantage that it lasts until your lashes grow out and are replaced with new ones, which normally takes between five and six weeks, and tinted eyelashes do not run in the water. It really does make an enormous difference to your holiday, and most salons now take no more than about fifteen minutes to do it.

WHEN YOU ARE THERE

So you are there, sitting in the sun having just arrived from cloudy England.

The secret to achieving a good tan without getting burnt is the care you take in the first few days. Unless you are dark-skinned, you must be careful during the first two or three days about the length of time you sit in the sun. Remember also that it is not just sitting in the sun; even when sitting in the shade, reflected sun can be just as burning.

If you are fair and have just arrived in a very hot climate, it is best not to sunbathe at all at the beginning. If the sun is not too strong, say the South of France in June or September, you can be more relaxed. If you took the precaution of having sun-lamp treatment before going away, you can be guided by the colour of your skin: you will find that the melanin will come to the surface almost immediately and give the protection you need.

If you are dark, you do not have to be so careful: if you are sensible you will also have had some sun-lamp treatment before going away, and after two days in the sun, this should give you all the protection you need. But remember that the bony areas of your body such as your shoulders, nose, knees and ankles burn much more quickly than more fleshy areas, and need to be watched.

Women often forget that the sun is drying to their hair and will make it brittle. Because you do not feel any physical sensation when hair is getting too much exposure to sun, it is sensible to wear some form of scarf or hat. This is particularly important if you colour or bleach your hair, otherwise the sun will lift the colour.

As I have a fair skin, which takes about ten days to acclimatize to the sun, I take the view that if I am only going to be away for two weeks there is no point in risking burning just to tan for such a short time. I spend most of my time on the beach under an umbrella and usually wearing a hat. Unfashionable perhaps, but kinder to the skin and in many ways more comfortable.

It is essential to use sun creams and oils. Enormous developments have been made over the last fifteen years which have led to a great proliferation of products on the market, and to some extent have added to consumer confusion. Without spending hours reading the directions on each product, how do you know which is right for you? My husband complains that life is no longer what it was twenty years ago, when it was just a simple matter of buying a bottle of Ambre Solaire!

In fact, he is not quite right. The increase in the number and types of

Few people realize that sun reflected on snow is twice as burning as direct sunlight: when it it is combined with the cold winds which you get ski-ing, it calls for maximum protection to the face. If you are fair, the best type of product to use is a sunblock, with a high protection number, such as Estée Lauder's Sunblock or Roc's Total Protection Cream. For darker skins, you can use sun creams with lower protection numbers, such as Ambre Solaire or Uvitan.

You need to be particularly careful about protecting your nose, which will otherwise catch the sun badly. I always advise using a sunblock on the nose regardless of your skin type.

A short course of sun lamp treatment in a salon before you go can help prepare your face for the sun: best of all is the new Uvasun head and shoulders lamp.

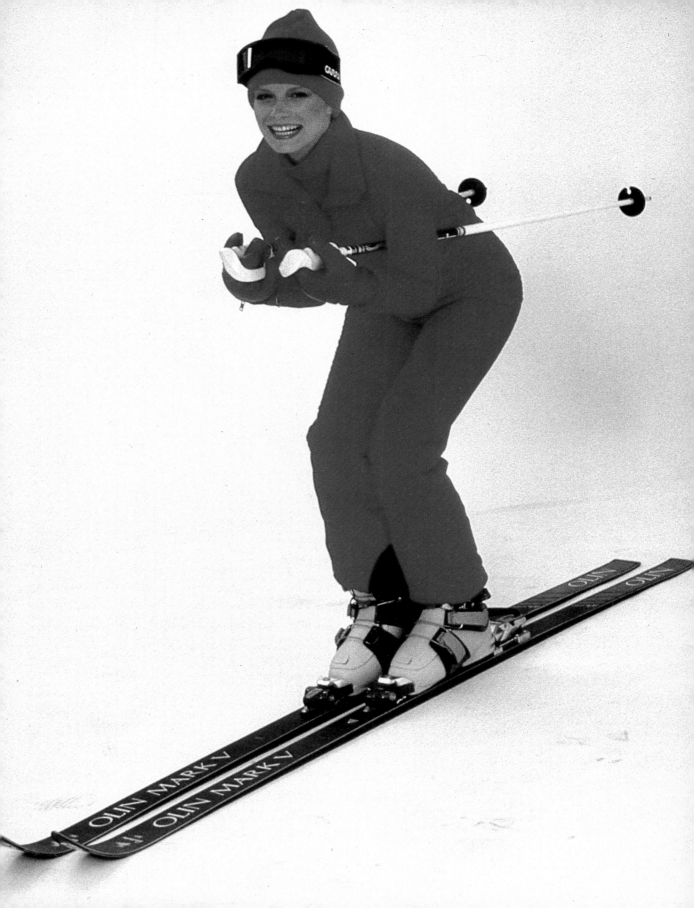

One way of keeping
cool in the sun : the idea
of spraying mineral
water on to your body
was first thought of by
models, who had to get
a deep, even tan quickly
for colour photography,
The cooling effect of the
water enabled them to
lie in the sun for longer.

For most of us there
are easier and more
comfortable ways of
getting a tan. Start with
a course of salon sun-
lamp treatments before
you go, and then ensure
you have the right sun
cream or oil when you
arrive.

It may take you a little
longer to get your tan,
but it is the sensible way
of doing it. I always find
it difficult to advise
women about which sun
product is best to use.
In the last few years,
most manufacturers
have followed each
other's latest product and
many products contain
the same protection
ingredients. Nearly
every year there is a
new one in fashion.
Currently the emphasis
is on including natural
ingredients, such as alo
cactus gel or coconut
oil.

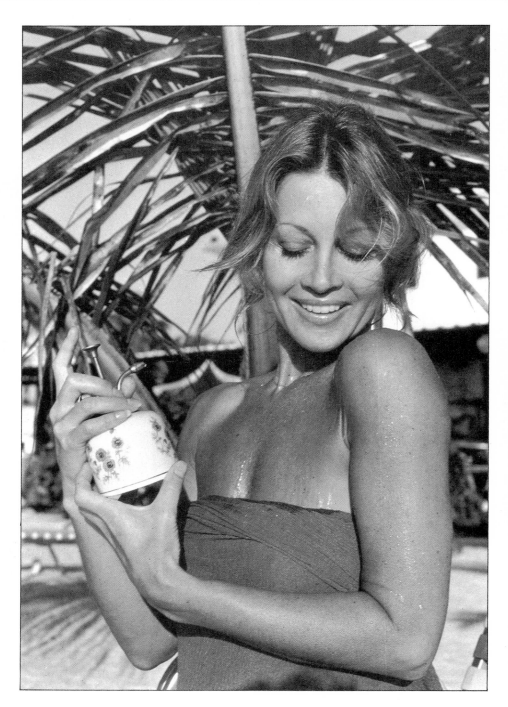

product on the market has led to more appropriate and effective products for each type of skin. The original Ambre Solaire my husband so fondly remembers was in fact an oil which browned and gave some protection to brown skins like his, but did not give much protection to the fairer northern skins.

If you know your way around the current products on the market, you can find ample protection for all types of skins in all types of situations.

Many manufacturers now number their products with a sun-rating factor from two to eight: this is intended as a guide to the amount of protection the product will give your skin. High numbers are more protective, low numbers less protective and will therefore tan you faster. Start with a higher number and after your skin has acclimatized to the sun you can move on to a lower number, the point being that since the high numbers are more protective they do not let the sun brown your skin so quickly. The lower numbers help to give you that really deep brown colour you see on models in advertisements.

To help confuse you further, sun products come in a variety of forms oil, gel, lotion, cream and milk. In general, the oils and gels tend to be at the lower numerical end of the product range, while the moisturized lotions and creams are in the higher numerical end. Creams and lotions with built-in moisturizers are best for treating dry skins, while light gels, oils and non-oily lotions will suit people with oily skins.

Most of the products on the market are in fact reasonably standard oils and creams with chemical screening agents such as para-amino benzoic acid, dihydroxy acetone or isobutylsalieyl cinnamate which filter out just enough of the burning ultra-violet rays to minimize sunburn, but allow enough rays through to give a tan in the shortest possible time. Recently there has been a return to natural anti-burn ingredients such as alo cactus gel and now coconut oil.

Most people will find that it takes them about four to five days to become fully acclimatized to the sun. After that you will find that a further forty-eight hours will achieve a really good tan, and from then on, the tan is unlikely to deepen to any real extent. How deeply you tan depends on your genes. Although each of us has the same number of melanocytes, the amount of melanin we produce varies.

Incidentally, sunbathing in the early morning or late afternoon almost never produces sunburn. When the sun is low in the sky, its radiation passes through a greater thickness of atmosphere. By the time the shorter wave lengths reach the earth most of their power has been decimated. The orange, yellow and red tints of sunrise and sunset are in fact the longer waves of light and are the safe end of the spectrum for the human skin.

There are, of course, people who are allergic to the sun. What is not so generally known is that some medicinal drugs such as tranquillizers, anti-biotics, and anti-histamines and the contraceptive pill can make some of us much more allergic to the sun than we would normally be. If you do find that for one reason or another you have developed an allergy to the sun, there is no need to despair completely. Before you go away, you can get yourself a fake tan, and when you arrive in the sun use a barrier-type sun cream which gives total protection.

If You Get Burned

If in spite of all your precautions you still find yourself with a reddened skin after your first day on the beach, do not make the mistake of applying cooling astringent lotions. Although they may feel wonderfully fresh, they contain alcohol and in fact will only make matters worse. Your skin's best friend on these occasions is the richest moisturizing cream or lotion that you have available: most of the sun protection ranges now sell very good after-tan lotions and creams which contain skin-moisturizing ingredients. In my experience one of the most effective of these is Alo After Tan which is part of a not very widely distributed range; it is made from the gel of the alovera cactus which has an immediate soothing effect on sun-reddened skins.

In an emergency you can also use a home-made remedy of kitchen ingredients. Mix the lightly beaten white of an egg with a little olive oil, and apply this to your skin.

Keeping Your Tan

Nothing looks better or more effective than a shiny suntanned body coming out of the water, but the effect is achieved far less naturally than you think.

Jet-set girls know all the tricks of how to water-proof their make-up and prepare their bodies for the hot sun, using sun lamps, sun screens, sun filters and even fake tans.

Many people ask for advice on how to preserve their tan. After all, if you have spent time, trouble and money in acquiring it, you do not want to throw it away.

In particular, those of us who are fair will find that our skin is inclined to peel: make sure you use plenty of moisturizing lotions and bath oils to act against the drying effect of bath water. In fact bathing, the action of soap and the friction of bath towels are the main destroyers of a tan. Bubble baths are another culprit as the detergent dries your skin, so leads to peeling.

The most effective way to prolong your tan is to oil your skin before bathing. Certainly do not lie soaking in hard water. In many ways a shower is better from this point of view than a bath. Do not rub yourself too hard with a towel afterwards. Invest in sun-lamp treatments to boost

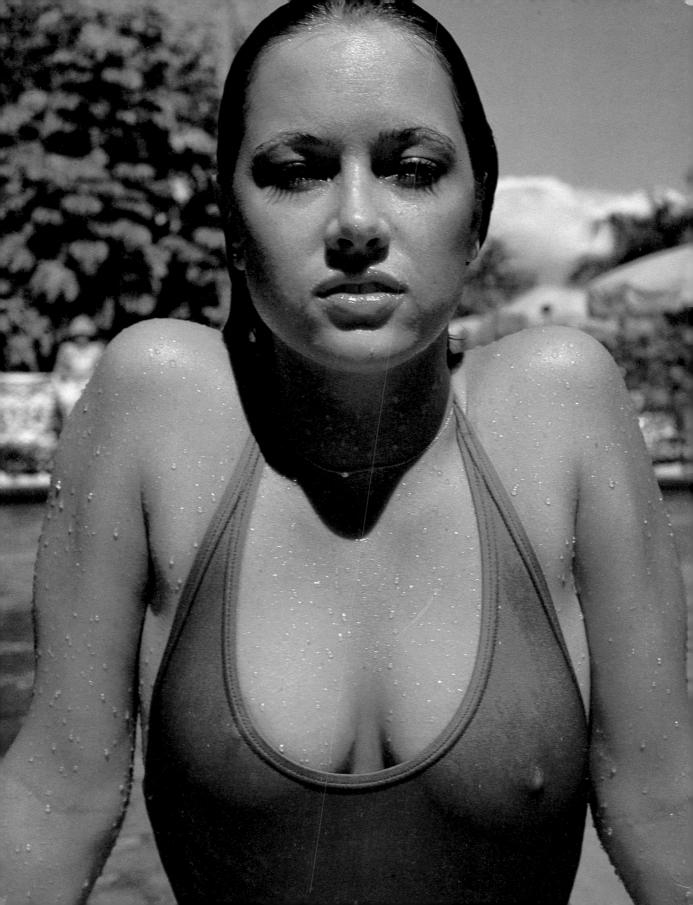

the colour as it begins to fade. The new UVA sunlamps will help preserve the colour and give you more mileage.

Make-up for the Sun and the Sea
The growing sophistication of life on the beach or by the swimming pool has meant that even when we have come straight out of the water, we still wish to look our best and most attractive. Nothing damages your confidence more than to come out of the sea or pool in some smart Mediterranean resort, being eyed by all those men, knowing that your mascara and make-up is running all down your face. It is really not a satisfactory solution to leave off your make-up, particularly if you are fair like me; this is not a moment one wants to look like an albino.

Not everyone is aware of the value of water-proof make-up. This was originally developed for film stars: they were soaked to the skin, wept, went deep-sea diving – and their cosmetics had to survive without running, smudging or streaking. For instance, any actress who wore block mascara would have found that it ran when she had to cry, so the forerunner of the water-proof cream mascara wands which all the beauty firms make today was the cream mascara in a tube which was oil-based and so water-resistant.

If you are going to look your best in the sun, go for a polished-looking face: a normal tinted foundation and tan-coloured powder look very made-up in bright sunlight, so try using a transparent bronze-tinted gel instead. If you have not used one of these before do not be startled because it looks like Marmite when it comes out of the tube; it will actually give a clear, golden tone to the skin, and will be virtually water-proof. These transparent bronze tans are really fake tans, and can be used all over your body as well as on your face. Unlike the so-called overnight tans, these fake tans wash off at will, but they are stable enough not to run when you swim. This type of skin colouring traces its history back to the walnut juice or solution of potassium permanganate crystals, which actors used to wear for a realistic-looking tan. Today's products are normally made from burnt sugar, in fact the ingredient in gravy browning.

To complement your shiny face you should switch to a shiny eye make-up: nothing is worse than matt-looking eyes with a shiny face. Nearly all make-up ranges today contain eye glosses, pearlized gels, pomades and polishers. They are better than powder or cream shadows because they are water-based and will not go into little lines in the crease of the eye. The pearl ingredient also gives a soft, light-reflecting colour to the lids that is ideal for an unpowdered summer face.

Some makes are shinier than others, and older eyes should avoid the shiniest as they tend to highlight wrinkles. Use one of the new soft-textured eye crayons instead; they are easy to use if you blend them carefully and the waxy texture makes them really lasting. Do not rely on any paint-on-with-water eyeliner or mascara: cake eyeliners and the old-fashioned block mascaras will run if eyelids and lashes get wet. The most water-proof you can use are liquid eyeliners that look like wand mascaras, and come ready to apply with a fine brush. If you really want to be up-to-date use kohl or a soft black crayon as an outline inside the rims of the eyes: water will not affect it.

As discussed in the section Before You Go, have your eyelashes tinted. This is a valuable alternative to wearing mascara on holiday, as it gives completely water-proof, smudge-proof colour to lashes.

Finish off the polished, shiny look by wearing one of the glossy-looking lipsticks in clear, transparent colours: they look super in summer and are ideal for wearing in and out of the water. Many of the new darker brown and rust-toned lipstick colours look good with a tan, especially with plenty of lip gloss over the top. Those skins which tan easily have the problem that the lipstick colours tend to lose their tone because of the amount of pigment in their skins; for them, clear coral shades are easily the best answer.

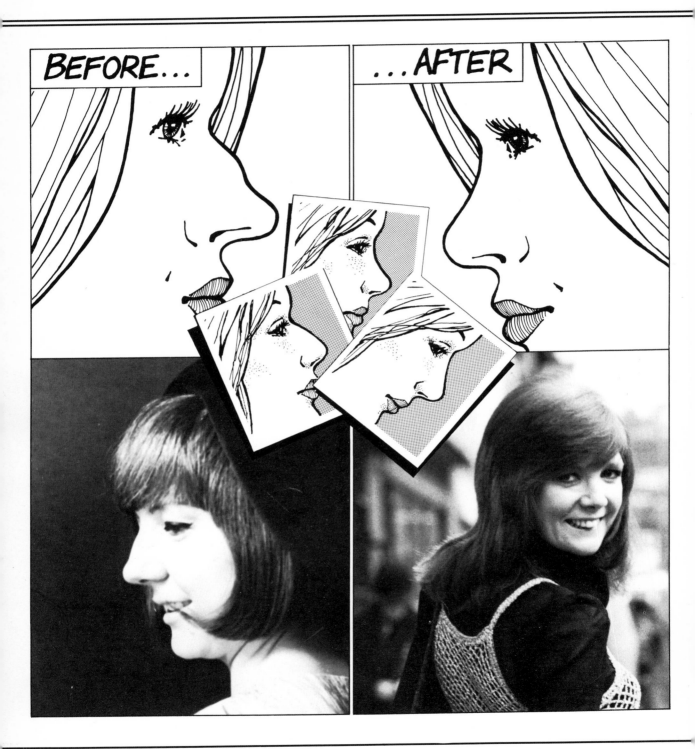

COSMETIC SURGERY

Plastic surgery is a subject which, when it comes up at a dinner party, is guaranteed to cause more controversy than any other aspect of beauty. Men almost invariably seem to take a very puritanical attitude; but then as I have said earlier in the book, most men are horrified if they hear that you wear more than lipstick and powder. The fact is that many women wish to improve their appearance and to get rid of obvious signs of ageing.

The interest in plastic surgery has grown tremendously in the last thirty years. At the end of the war there were approximately 15,000 registered operations a year in Britain for surgery for cosmetic reasons. Today the number is nearly 750,000. No longer is it just the rich and privileged who have this type of operation.

There is nothing new about the idea of using surgery to improve the appearance. For centuries Indian doctors have used skin grafts for improving deformed or damaged noses and ears, and many of their early skills are still used today. However, it was the Second World War that really advanced the skills of plastic surgery.

Much of the work which is done today in this country was pioneered in the war by two leading surgeons at East Grinstead hospital, Gilles and McIndoe, to help heal the dreadful burns and scars of the Battle of Britain fighter pilots.

Every year, as new skills and safeguards are developed, the number of operations performed for cosmetic reasons increases. New techniques in stitching have been developed to minimize scars, and modern antibiotics have cut down the risk of infection, so less time need be spent in hospital.

For most people the main problem is how to set about getting something done, and it is still true to say that in Britain most surgeons prefer using their skills to repair damage caused in accidents or to correct malformations

Changing the shape of your nose is the most obvious example of a cosmetic surgery operation. Photographs are taken by the surgeon to show the different shapes available to their client. Cilla Black's nose is no longer the dominant feature of her face; her eyes and bone structure now play a more important part than they did.

in children, than to operate on women who want to re-capture their youth. There still exists the old prejudice that too much concern with your looks is simply vanity.

There are basically two ways of finding a surgeon to perform a cosmetic operation. As most people know, all surgeons who are Fellows of the Royal College of Surgeons are governed by a strict code of conduct. They are not allowed to advertise, and just as if you wish to have the services of a barrister you have to go through a solicitor, so with a surgeon you must go through a GP. Unfortunately many women are shy about discussing with their family doctor the reasons why they want cosmetic surgery; also, some GPs have strong views about cosmetic surgery and feel that it is a flippant whim of a woman to want to have it.

If you are up against these views, one answer to the problem of finding a surgeon is to ring any of the big London teaching hospitals, who will usually give you the names and addresses of their consultant plastic surgeons. Once you have this information you may find it easier to talk to your doctor about having an operation. He will see that you are serious about it and he is likely to be much more understanding.

The alternative way of having the operation is to go to one of the special cosmetic surgery clinics. There has been a rapid growth in the number of these clinics in the last few years, partly as an answer to the increasing interest in face lifts. They are staffed with a full team of anaesthetists, surgeons and GPs, thereby overcoming the problem of going to your family doctor. However standards do vary.

My own feeling about these clinics is that the really good ones do fulfil a role, namely that some people are much happier having a cosmetic operation in a place which is exclusively geared to this type of work, and where there is no feeling of taking up valuable nursing time when there are seriously ill people elsewhere as in a general hospital. But if you decide to go to one of them, I would advise you to be careful about checking on the surgeon.

These clinics employ and use Fellows of the Royal College of Surgeons, but they are not always what are called "accredited plastic surgeons". I have heard of cases where there has been a botched job, because the surgeon has not been a specialist in cosmetic work. Do not forget that it is perfectly legal for an operation for, say, a new nose, to be performed by a dental surgeon. This is why I believe it is so important to establish that the surgeon who is going to perform the operation is fully experienced in cosmetic work. As I have discussed earlier in this chapter, one of the great difficulties for a member of the general public is the lack of information that is available on how to find the right surgeon who will do a really good job.

I asked a leading member of the British Association of Plastic Surgeons why it was that they did not run some form of advisory service which would enable people to obtain the names of their accredited members. Although he was very sympathetic to my views, he still thought that it was desirable always to have a professional recommendation from your doctor, who after all is familiar with your medical history.

Cosmetic surgery operations fall into two main categories: those to change your looks and those to prevent signs of ageing. The most usual and obvious example of an operation to improve your looks is that to change the shape of your nose. The art of nose surgery has improved enormously in recent years, and I am continually surprised at the amazing transformation that this operation can make to people's appearance. The nose is a focal point of the face, and a large bulbous nose can dominate any face. I know that if I had been born with one, I would certainly have a nose operation today. Nearly all the people who have had one are unanimous in their pleasure from having had the operation.

One of the intriguing and successful results of having a nose operation is that the person often forgets afterwards her nose has ever been a problem. One woman said, "I never think of my nose any more, in fact now I wonder whether it was really as awful as I once imagined it was!"

The operation is called rhinoplasty, and in my view requires maximum cosmetic experience on the part of the surgeon whose creative ability will be called upon to give you a well-balanced result.

As with all types of plastic surgery, before and after photographs are an important part of the process. At first consultation pictures will be taken full face, three-quarter face, and profile. Some surgeons will also take a plaster cast of your existing nose and show you casts of their proposed variation. Others use X-ray pictures of the cartilage and bone formation inside the nose, which are teamed with a black and white photograph of the outside of your nose: in this way the surgeon can show you how he plans to reform the nose and is better able to judge the thickness of the skin, which can often be responsible for a lot of unnecessary bulk on the nose.

Obviously a nose that will suit one person is not going to be quite right for anyone else, therefore every case has to be studied individually. Considerations such as facial expressions, movement of features, age, height and general build of the patient have to be studied. For instance, it would be impossible to imagine General de Gaulle with a small nose or Twiggy with a long one.

Remember too that a nose only attains its major growth by the age of seventeen. Because the face is still changing until it reaches maturity in the early twenties, most surgeons are unlikely to agree to perform a nose operation on a teenager.

Correcting noses that are too large or too long, too short or noticeably crooked, straightening a nose which is hooked or bulbous at the tip, are all possibilities with modern facial surgery. In almost all cases operations are performed from the inside of the nose through the nostrils, so that there is no external scarring. The surgeon separates the skin from the underlying bone and cartilage and uses miniature surgical instruments to cut and remove excess bone and cartilage. Occasionally it is necessary to build up a depression in the nose, in which case a bit of cartilage will be taken from behind the ear, or bone from, say, the hip.

The final step is to pack out the nose with surgical wadding before applying a small splint and bandage. Most patients say it is uncomfortable rather than very painful, similar to a heavy cold in terms of soreness and breathing, and frequently the eyes are swollen and bruised. The stay in hospital for this operation is usually about a week, but it is sometimes possible to go home after four or five days wearing the splint. This is usually removed after a week. The results of this operation are permanent.

I sometimes see women who have had their nose operated on and are very worried as to whether or not it has been a success. In most cases they come to discuss make-up as soon as the bruising has disappeared, which is frequently only two or three weeks after having the operation. But with most nose operations a certain amount of facial swelling can remain for up to three months, and it is important to allow the re-shape to settle down before judging the final success of the operation.

Correcting bat ears is an operation which is sometimes recommended for children and teenagers. Although the rest of their face can take much longer to develop, children's ears are fully grown by the time they are eight or nine. Excessively large protruding ears can be a real trial for a young person, although the current preference for wearing hair much longer has meant that they are not the problem they were twenty years ago.

During the operation, which lasts about an hour, incisions are made behind the ears and the surgeon remodels the cartilage in the ears themselves and stitches them back into place closer to the head. Bandages are necessary for four to five days and sometimes patients are required to wear a light bandage around the head when going to bed at night for a few months after the operation. Special care is taken to make all incisions in the crevices and folds of the ears so that there is no risk of scarring. Again the results are permanent.

The two most common operations to combat ageing are those to remove bags under the eyes and a full face lift.

A full face lift is a big operation: incisions are made in the hair above the temples, going down in front of the ears, under the lobes and ending behind the ears. Very little hair needs to be cut; bandaging is light and only lasts for about forty-eight hours after the operation. Most patients feel dopey and uncomfortable, but are not in any real pain. Stitches are removed after a week.

The main improvements achieved with a full face lift are in smoothing cheeks, getting rid of nose to mouth lines, giving a firmer jaw line and improving the appearance of the throat.

Whether you decide you need to have surgery at all will depend largely on your bone structure and to some extent your skin type. Eye operations are more likely to be suitable for people with fine, dry skins, who are more prone to lines and wrinkles, particularly around the eyes. Full face lifts are more appropriate for women with small features whose bone structure is not very prominent. If you have strong features – a big chin, well-defined cheekbones – you will find that you keep your facial contours better than women with small features, and you will therefore be less likely to need a full face lift.

One fact that is not generally realized is that a face lift is not permanent. This is one reason why some surgeons may not agree to do a lift if they feel that the patient is too young and the skin and contours are not sufficiently wrinkled or sagging. There is no perfect age for a face lift; the result would usually be less dramatic with a woman in her late forties than with someone, say, in her sixties. It is, however, possible to have more than one lift; the original scars can be cut out when the next incisions are made and a second operation need not be as extensive as the first.

Eye bags are caused by little hernias of fat that get trapped in the delicate tissues underneath the eyes and these usually become more noticeable when wrinkles come with ageing. The operation to remove the bags and wrinkles is done under a general anaesthetic and takes about one to one and a half hours (some continental surgeons use local anaesthetics, but most English surgeons I have spoken to say the injections can cause puffiness). Because the incisions are made very close to the edge of the eyes, under the lower lashes, the line of stitches is almost invisible.

Eyes are kept lightly bandaged for twenty-four hours but there is very little discomfort. As the skin around the eyes heals quickly, the slight bruising and swelling last only for a few days. In fact most people find it can quite easily be camouflaged with foundation, or by wearing tinted glasses. Stitches are removed in ten days, but even then you should be a bit careful

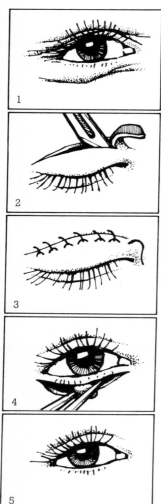

To remove drooping
eyelids (1): surplus skin
is removed from the
crease of the lid (2);
the cut is stitched (3);
to eliminate bags,
fatty tissue is removed
close to the bottom
lashes (4); eyes look
younger with all bags
gone (5).

about wearing mascara straight away as the oil-based colour can get into the scars and cause puffiness.

Heavy eyelids, which give eyes a hooded look, can be removed by the same operation: in this case incisions are made in the creases of the eyes, surplus loose skin is removed and scars are effectively hidden.

There are also specialized surgical remedies for small lines and furrows, notably on the forehead, around the eyes and at the edge of the top lip. A French treatment called "threading" is a good way of treating these small lines. It is done under a local anaesthetic – a threaded needle is inserted at one end of the wrinkle and drawn out at the other. Both ends of the thread are knotted. Because the thread is alien to the body, fibrous tissue builds up over it, but under the skin thus plumping out the wrinkle, which will either disappear or lessen in depth. When this healing process has taken place, after about ten to fourteen days, the knots are cut and the threads withdrawn. This is particularly suitable for the longer furrows on the forehead.

Another method of line filling is galvanopuncture. This is done with an electric needle and causes a little burn in the base of a skin furrow, thus swelling it out, and is particularly suitable for little lines, such as those which appear round the edge of the lips.

A third method which is sometimes used for lip furrows, but which is mainly used for dealing with acne scars, is dermabrasion. Spots and skin eruptions which are a feature of acne are infections caused by blocked oil ducts. The longer the ducts in the skin, the more prone they are to infection. Dermabrasion planes the skin and so shortens the ducts, allowing the growth of a finer-pored skin.

The surgeon uses a general anaesthetic, and an electrically operated abrasive disc or brush which is about the size of a five pence piece. Depending on the severity of the problem the process of planing the skin may take an hour or just a few minutes. Antibiotics are used to promote healing and bandages are worn for about twenty-four hours. Once the bandages are removed the scab begins to form on the face which is treated with ointment to keep it soft; a few days later a special solution is used several times a day until after about ten days the scab comes off. The new skin looks red and sunburnt, but resumes its normal colour quite quickly. Anyone who has had this operation always has to be very careful of exposing the face to the sun, as it can give a mottled uneven effect to the skin pigment. A girl I know well in her mid-thirties, who had a skin which was troubled by acne for many years with the consequent scars, had this operation. It completely changed the texture and behaviour of her skin by shortening the ducts, and today she has a clear and much finer-pored skin.

There is an alternative operation to dermabrasion, which is a chemical peel with phenol. This is a form of carbolic acid and gives the skin a second degree burn. In my opinion this can cause a number of unpleasant side effects, since the chemical can be absorbed through the skin. Most cosmetic surgeons that I have spoken to do not approve of this method of promoting skin peeling and reckon that dermabrasion is just as effective, with considerably less risk to the body.

Another growing area of cosmetic surgery are operations to improve body shape. Today when it is fashionable to wear the kind of clothes that reveal the body, it is quite understandable that physical defects can cause women genuine unhappiness. Sometimes I am asked, usually by men, "Why on earth do people have body surgery?" Basically the reason is that because of childbirth and sometimes obesity, the skin can stretch until it is several sizes too large for the frame inside it. When this has happened there is only one way of dealing with this problem, which is to tailor one to fit the other with surgery. Certainly the after effects of child-bearing can cause special problems, and no one wants to feel doomed to live for the rest of her life with shrunken breasts, sagging abdomen, and a flabby waist-line.

One of the most popular body operations is for correcting sagging breasts, and a number of different materials have been tried for improving the shape of the breasts. Among the substances experimented with have been liquid and gel silicones, and a spongy substance called polyethylene. A bag with one of these substances is slipped into the breasts with only a small incision, leaving a tiny scar. Most incisions are made below the curve of the breast or sometimes diagonally at the sides in order to maintain the rounded symmetrical shape.

One of the big advantages of the newest implants with the silicone gel is that the body's own tissue fibres can grow into the implant, and there is a self-adherent quality to the gel which ensures that it will not travel round the body. One of the main problems of the early operations using liquid silicone was that it could move, and sometimes turned up in quite large quantities in different areas of the body. There were also instances where the silicone hardened and went lumpy. Happily, liquid silicone is now no longer allowed to be used.

There is also an operation for reducing the size of the bust, where surplus tissue is removed from under the curve of the breast. It is sometimes even necessary to re-position the nipples which can be done with a skin graft.

Both operations for breast surgery require a stay in hospital of about a week, mainly because it is necessary to make sure that no excess fluid remains: a small tube is left in for draining purposes after the operation and is

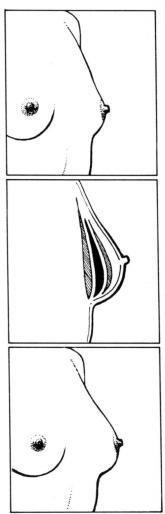

The shape and size of small breasts can now be improved. In the middle picture a pouch containing silicone gel is inserted into the breast in front of or between the pectoral muscles to give the natural-looking fullness shown in the third picture.

	Recommended Age	Operation Time	Stay in Hospital	Convalescence	Approximate Cost including Hospitalization	Duration of Results
FACE LIFT	45+	2–2½ hrs.	3–4 days	2–3 weeks	£750–£1200	8–10 yrs.
EYELIDS upper & lower	30+	1 hour	24 hrs.	1 week to 10 days	£450–£750	10–15 yrs.
NOSE RE-SHAPE	17+	45 mins. to 1 hour	4–5 days	2–3 weeks	£450–£1000	Permanent
BUST INCREASE	20+	1 hour	2–3 days	10 days	£800–£1000	Permanent
BUST REDUCTION	18+	2 hours	1 week	2–3 weeks	£750–£1400 (sometimes available on Nat. Health)	15–20 yrs.
CORRECTING BAT EARS	6+	1 hour	24 hrs.	10 days	£450–£750	Permanent
STOMACH IMPROVING	25+	1½ hrs.	1 week	2–3 weeks	Allow £1500	Permanent (unless patient becomes obese)

What you want to know about cosmetic operations.

removed after forty-eight hours. Most patients who have breast operations are delighted with the results. The two most usual reasons for having this operation are to improve the shape of sagging breasts after childbirth, and enlarge small breasts.

It is still impossible to remove stretch marks caused by carrying children or obesity, although flabby tissue, which can be unsightly and uncomfortable, can be cut out and tidied up. The scar is left low down across the stomach so that it is possible to wear a bikini or two-piece swimsuit without it showing. This operation, called abdominal lipectomy, takes longer and patients are usually in hospital for about ten days to two weeks. A flabby spare tyre which is due to dieting can also be cut out, but this scar is much more difficult to hide.

Successful operations are also carried out to remove slack-looking skin underneath the tops of the arms and to improve the shape of thighs which have become flabby. But it is important to realize that you will be left with scars; although these can be hidden on the insides of arms and legs, it is essential to weigh up the pros and cons before you decide to have it done. People who have had arm operations say that they find their clothes look much better and somehow the fact that they no longer have folds of loose skin in such an easily seen place makes them much less self-conscious.

Unfortunately, very little can be done to slim down heavy-looking legs around the ankles. It is a difficult area on which to operate, because of all the muscles, blood vessels (particularly if there is any tendency to varicose veins) and lymphatic glands. Apart from being very costly, requiring a lot of physiotherapy and after care, scarring is the real problem.

One of the important things which most doctors want to know when you go to discuss cosmetic surgery is what your motivations are for having the operation. It is very important to realize that surgeons are not miracle workers and they do not like operating on the type of patient who has an unreal image of herself and wants to look completely different. Patients who arrive for a consultation with pictures of movie stars who are considerably younger than themselves, or who are pinning all their hopes on saving a failing marriage by having cosmetic surgery, are obviously discouraged. Most surgeons agree that simple vanity is the best motive for cosmetic surgery.

This is not to say that many people will not experience tremendous psychological benefits from the correction of a minor abnormality, such as a large nose which has troubled them all their lives. Certainly the psychological boost which women can get from an operation to remove signs of ageing such as getting rid of bags under the eyes, or a sagging jaw line, can be tremendous. As one of them said to me, "Knowing I look better makes me feel ten years younger, and it is so marvellous that my friends don't keep telling me that I am looking tired".

Most cosmetic surgery is not available on the National Health, unless the fault is so severe as to cause evident psychological distress. Even then, there can be a long waiting list and in most cases accident victims and children are given priority. Nor will the medical insurance companies, such as BUPA or Private Patients Plan, cover your costs unless the surgery has become necessary as the result of an accident. Improving your looks with plastic surgery will cost you money, therefore, but it is nearly always worth it.

However much time and trouble you take over your make-up and skin care, all will be wasted if you neglect your hair. Nothing affects your looks as much as your hair, and this becomes increasingly true as you get older.

Today, when there are so many popular and famous hairdressers, it is difficult for us to realize that in the thirties there were only four top names in hairdressing and they all worked within a small radius in Mayfair. Antoine was the best known: a Paris hairdresser who rented Lord Salisbury's town house in Dover Street, he cut the Duchess of Windsor's hair and had a glass coffin in his home that created a sensation. On the other side of the street was Vasco: this was a family business and the family was responsible for the original Bubbles style. Emile was originally in Conduit Street and did the Royal Family's hair. Phyllis Earle was in Dover Street specializing in colouring. A distinctive touch of this salon was that it collected new pound notes from the bank every day, so that ladies would not have to handle dirty money!

Hairdressing, as we know it now, really took off as a business after the war. It is interesting that of all the post-war hairdressers, only Raymond appears to have worked for one of the pre-war big four. He left Vasco to open his own salon in Grafton Street in 1938, and Alan Spiers, Xavier and Robert Fielding all worked with him before starting up on their own.

The fifties were good years for hairdressing: customers were plentiful, if not all "U" in Nancy Mitford's new social terminology. As one hairdresser explained, "Before the war nearly all our clients were county and society women. People from the suburbs or even business girls who worked in London never came into the salons. In the fifties, hairdressing started to become much less of a class thing, you began to get models, secretaries, starlets and even charabanc tours, as well as the socialites and debs."

Salons were remodelled: cubicles disappeared and were replaced by open planning, with dressing-tables, wash-basins and drying-bays – which accommodated twice the number of customers. Raymond appeared on television and demonstrated his new Penny Bun style, and became known to a wide audience as Mr Teazy-Weazy. Hundreds of women, who had

Vidal Sassoon's famous sixties creation, the Five Point Bob. Inset, we show the style being cut.

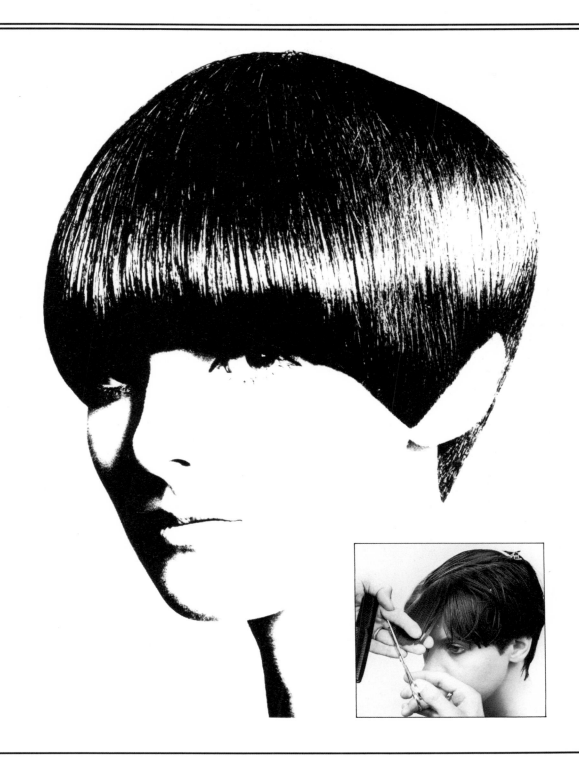

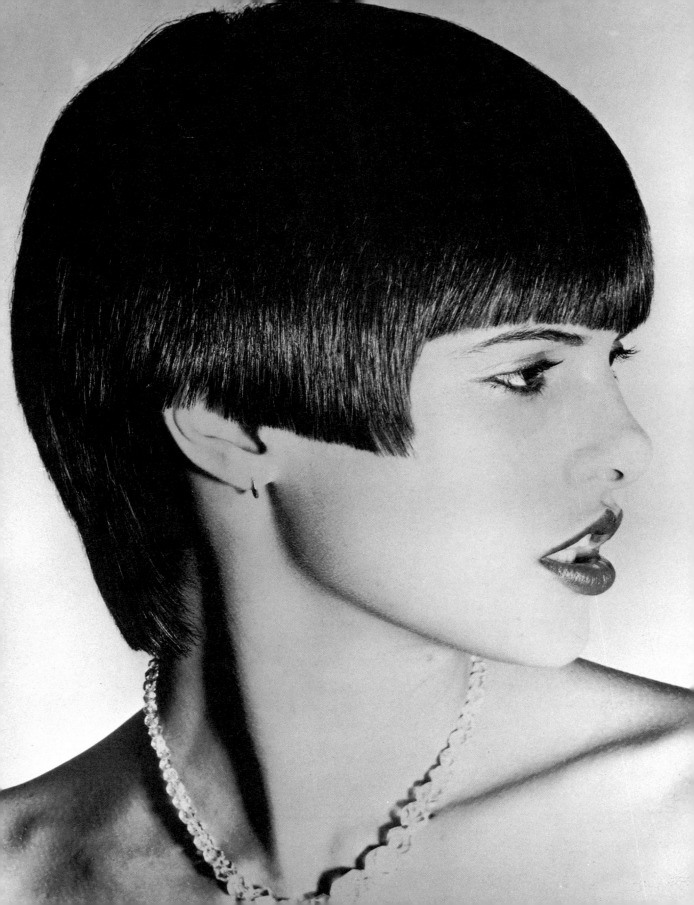

never thought of having their hair done in the West End before, flocked to Grafton Street. New salons sprouted to meet the new demand, and although a number of them were in Mayfair, there were also many in residential areas.

This was the era of that extraordinary phenomenon, the fantasy hairstyle competition. I have always failed to see its relevance to life, in that it is inconceivable that anyone with any sense of style would have wanted to wear hair in such a way. Almost invariably, the fantasy hairstyles were executed on platinum blond hair, as darker hair colouring did not show up the elaborate swirls and curls: as if this was not enough, the blond hair was rinsed in delicate shades of lilac, pink and blue, and back-combed and lacquered into a consistency which achieved the effect of candy floss.

In his book, *Sorry to Keep You Waiting, Madam*, Vidal Sassoon describes his early years in hairdressing and the fever which gripped hairdressers in those days to create fantasy styles which, as he says, "might never be seen in public". Three or four thousand hairdressers would turn up to watch. But at least they gave an impetus, which should not be underestimated, to a young thrusting business.

Some salons seemed to encourage more talent than others, and they were not always the best known. In the early fifties, Romaines, a salon in the Edgware Road, London, which was still in business until recently, had half a dozen budding top names working there before they moved on to open up on their own. They included Vidal Sassoon, Harold Leighton, Leon Freeman, who opened with David Sandler, and Gerard Austen, who first ran Carita and then later joined Vidal Sassoon.

As so often happens, a particularly successful salon spawns a new wave of young hairdressers. Probably the most successful ex-Vidal stylist was Leonard who set up on his own with Raphael as a partner in the late fifties. Although the partnership did not last very long, Leonard continued on his own and attracted a great deal of hairdressing talent. As he always says, "I am training my future opposition all the time", and sure enough there are now at least five salons started by ex-Leonard stylists dotted around London. Names like Michaeljohn, Stafford and Frieda, Colombe and Neville Daniel have opened mainly in the last few years. Most are situated a good mile from Leonard.

It is now a normally accepted rule that you do not set up just round the corner from your ex-boss's shop. But ever since the first great exodus of Vidal stylists, of whom Leonard was one, most of the top crimpers have been much more relaxed about the rules which used to be part of every successful hairdresser's employment contract. Among the many trends set by Vidal, he relaxed the attitude towards employees leaving to start their

This eighties version of Vidal Sassoon's classic geometric hairstyle is cut with a new precision layering technique by Herta Keller, their European Artistic Director. In his book *Sorry to Keep You Waiting Madam*, Vidal gives much of the credit for the inspiration for geometric cutting to Mary Quant; "I decided to cut hair the way Mary cuts material, no fuss, no ornamentation, just a neat, clean swinging line." Like all Sassoon cuts, this one follows the basic skull structure and natural line of hair growth so that the style will shake back into place. It is a natural successor to his famous early sixties creations such as the Five Point Cut, Short Back and Long Sides and the Asymmetric Cut.

own business. He understood that a good young ambitious person could not be held for ever.

One of the most important trends in the last fifteen years has been the way in which Mayfair hairdressers have spread out more and more into the provinces. Raymond has franchized salons all over the country; ever since he appeared on television in the fifties as Mr Teazy-Weazy, he has been a household name and personality. André Bernard were the first to turn their hairdressing business into a quoted company on the stock exchange, and are said to have made more money in the out-of-London branches than in Mayfair. Vidal Sassoon expanded his business in a way never previously imagined. Except for a brief period in the thirties when Antoine from Paris had his salon in Mayfair, hairdressing had not crossed international boundaries in the way that Helena Rubinstein and Elizabeth Arden had done with their beauty salons and products. Vidal in the last ten years has gone to America, taken it by storm, even has his own TV chat show, has salons all over America, and his hair products are now one of the leading hair-care brands there.

Styles of decor in salons have changed almost as much as hairstyling itself. After the war anyone who left a salon and set up on his own automatically recreated the gilded chandelier style of his ex-employer, and usually used a French adaptation of his name. Change came suddenly in the sixties with names such as Crimpers and Smile, whose salons reflected the directness and appropriateness of their names.

As in all walks of life, expensive does not automatically mean best, and obviously not all expensive hairdressers are good; some will be past their best. But as long as you keep in touch with the names you see in magazines and talk to fashion-conscious friends, you should not go far wrong. In my experience, in hairdressing, expensive is more likely to mean best than in many other fields. There are a number of reasons which are worth mentioning. Top hairdressing is very much a chicken and egg situation: top hairdressers do magazine work, which keeps them in touch with the latest fashion ideas and styles; in turn, they attract celebrities as part of their clientele; they stimulate the hairdressers to keep ahead in their styling and not unnaturally the most ambitious, talented young stylists want to work for those at the top.

I certainly practise what I preach, and have always been prepared to pay for a good cut. But a word of warning. There is no point in going to a good hairdresser if you are going to tell him or her exactly how you want your hair cut. My observation is that most women tend to hang on to their old styles for too long, in the same way that they continue to use lipsticks long

A smooth shoulder-length bob of shining hair; the kind of style that looks good on almost all types of hair. It is cut and styled by Vidal Sassoon's Artistic Director Christopher Brooker, who has added an eighties touch to the style with the slim-rolled braid of hair that holds the hair back at one side. Skilful cutting like this can make thin, straight hair look thicker as well as making thick, bushy hair look sleeker and more manageable.

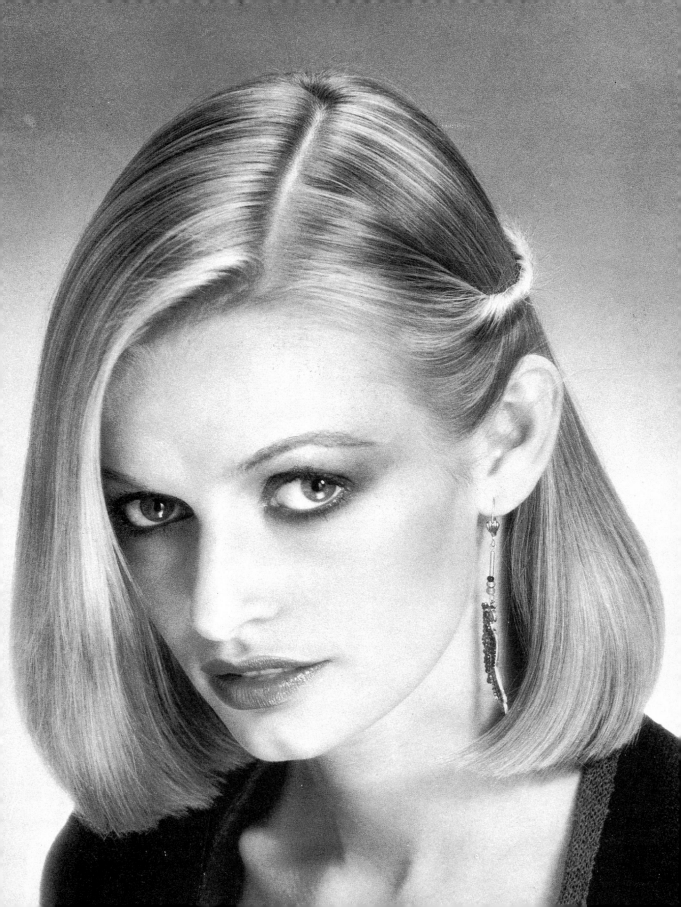

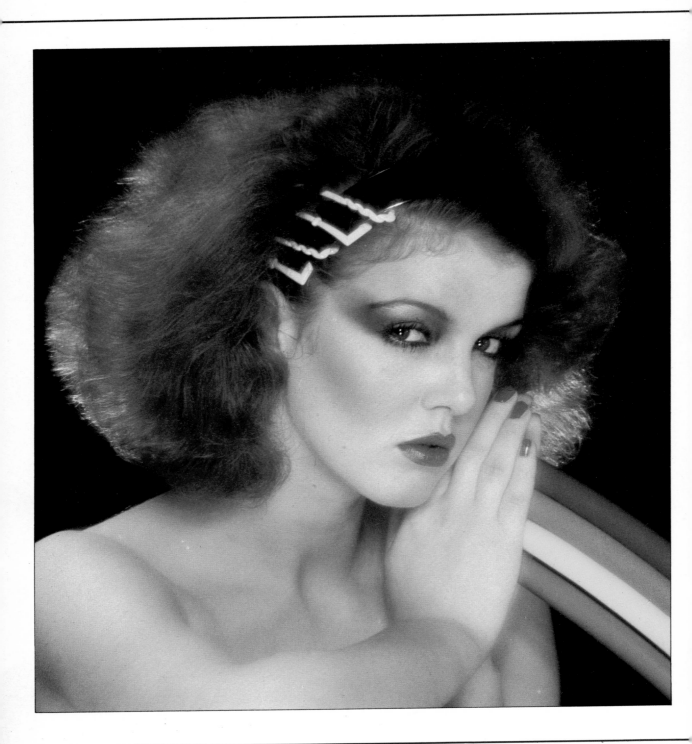

after the colour has gone out of fashion. Remember that hairdressers are more in touch with the trends than you are. This does not mean that you will automatically like the cut that you get from every good hairdresser, or that there are no good hairdressers locally; of course there are. But unless you have already found one, you have a much greater chance of satisfaction if you go to a well-known hairdresser; at least you will get what you are paying for. If the cut is wrong there is sadly nothing you can do, except to wait for your hair to grow and then try someone else. Normally you will know straight away if the cut you have had is good, because your hair will keep its shape and be much easier to manage. If you do not find this, do not struggle on thinking that he or she will improve next time. This seldom happens. Do not worry about changing; hairdressers are used to it.

It is not entirely chance that so many women who have found the right hairdresser treat them as personal friends. Women know that nothing gives them more confidence than their hair looking right, so that the person who does it well becomes important.

Women are always asking whether I think men or women are the best hairdressers. My view is that it is very much a matter of opinion and personal preference, depending to some extent on your relationship with men and women. For instance, Bianca Jagger once told me, "I prefer a man to do my hair because I have a better relationship with men." So too Thea Porter, who says, "I find they are less temperamental than women and don't mind so much if you tell them something's wrong." Jill Bennett's view on the other hand is that, "I think I'd always go to a woman; on the whole I like women better than men," and added that she found her hairdresser has a very sympathetic personality.

I always go to a woman hairdresser for choice. I think a lot of men hairdressers see women as glamorous individuals and tend to give them the styles they think they ought to have, and are inclined to be more autocratic. A woman stylist knows the problems; she understands what it is like to go around feeling her hair is looking awful. You do not have to explain. She is more likely to listen to your point of view. Patricia at the Cadogan Club, a successful salon in the heart of residential Knightsbridge, says that in her view there is no real disadvantage in being a woman in hairdressing today. I also agree with Vidal that the whole business is now much more professional than it was. At one time you found men who were not really much good; they sent all their clients out with the same style and got away with it purely on the strength of their personalities. But there is no substitute for good professional cutting. It is not entirely coincidence that young girls, who used to be anti-hairdresser and wore their hair straight and hanging down

This bouffant, Afro-Look hairstyle is a good example of where make-up is influenced by the way you wear your hair; this style calls for a strong make-up with plenty of emphasis on eyes and lips to give balance to the whole effect. The hairstyle, with its pretty gilt ornament that emphasizes the line, was created by Harold Leighton for Essanelle and Mark Easton did the make-up.

The eye make-up colour was silvery grey (such as Estée Lauder's Deep Smoke and Silvery Grey Eye Colour Stick; or Princess Galitzine's Silvery Grey and Grey Eye pencils). Leichner's Silver Streak and Charles of the Ritz Softshine shadow Pommade also give this effect. It was complemented by a brilliant red lipstick (Elizabeth Arden International lipstick and matching nail polish).

to their shoulders until a few years ago, now realize the difference when their hair has been well cut.

Of all the money you spend on your looks, I firmly believe that the first priority is a good cut for your hair. If you spend enough on your cut, you will find that it is easy to keep your hair looking attractive. I would far rather have an expensive cut once every six weeks and look after my hair myself in the intervening period than go to a cheaper hairdresser for a "weekly do"; you can nearly always tell if hair has been expensively cut and styled.

Well-kept hair starts with professional shaping. A good hairstylist cuts hair according to its natural texture, such as fine or coarse, straight or curly, thick or thin. One of the basic reasons for badly cut hair is that the hair has been cut regardless of its basic type: you will find that it will not behave properly regardless of the amount of time you spend conditioning it.

The type of hair you have has been decided for you by your genes and it is up to you with professional help to make the most of what you have got. Sometimes women with fine straight hair wish they could find a conditioner that would make their hair more manageable; they want it to have the same body and bounce as someone who has thick coarse hair with a natural wave. They are asking for the impossible; the way your hair behaves is governed by the way in which it comes out of your head. Wavy hair grows at a slight angle and so is distorted into an oval shape, instead of being round like straight hair.

People sometimes think it is possible to make their hair grow long and faster by conditioning treatments, or by eating the right foods. Once again your individual rate of hair growth is governed by your genes. If you are one of those people who can never manage to grow her hair further than her shoulders and you envy your friend whose hair is long enough to sit on, it means that your growth pattern is different to hers, and no amount of conditioning or sensible eating will alter this fact. Everyone's hair stays on her head for between two to six years until it is pushed out by the formation of new hair in the root. If your hair will not grow any further than your shoulders, it means that the new growth is pushing it out more quickly than your friend's, whose hair is likely to stay on her head for longer.

HAIR TYPES

The most important point after your cut is to organize your hair routine, which will vary according to your hair type.

Dry Hair

This needs a mild shampoo: liquid cream shampoos, usually made with additives such as herbs, egg, beer or lanolin are best as they are not too degreasing. Lather once only so that the hair is not stripped of natural oils. Follow with a conditioning cream rinse or protein-structuring setting lotion. Because dry hair can be fine and is inclined to be thin, it is important to eat plenty of the kind of foods that help boost hair condition. Vitamin B, calcium salts, mineral salts and sulphur are good for hair and are available in natural form in wholemeal bread, brewer's yeast, wheat-germ and liver.

Oily Hair

Top priority should be given to cleansing, using two latherings (unless you wash your hair more than twice a week when one lathering is sufficient). Massage your scalp, moving it around with your fingers, do not rub, and avoid brushing as this stimulates oil flow. In our grandmothers' days when you had to fetch water to wash your hair and make a soap solution to clean it, it was less trouble to bring up the shine to your smooth classically styled tresses with 100 strokes of the hair brush, especially if it was performed by your maid, than to go to all the trouble of washing and drying your hair. But today, when some people shampoo their hair five or six times a week and wear the type of styles that need lift and bounce rather than smooth polish, brushing has become obsolete. Modern aerosol dry shampoos can be an alternative to over-frequent washing and are much finer and easier to use than they used to be. If you find it hard to get the dry shampoo out of your hair, force the teeth of your comb into a piece of cotton wool; comb your hair after spraying and the cotton wool will pick up the powder and surplus oil. Oily hair usually goes with an over-oily skin type, so it is best to avoid too many greasy and acid-forming foods such as chips, cakes, pastries, chocolate and shell fish.

Problem Hair

Dandruff and all forms of scalp scaliness are very commonplace complaints. Oily dandruff is usually a bacterial infection that goes with greasy hair and skin; medicated shampoos can be very effective for treating it. There is another type of dry scalp scaliness which is usually noticeable in smaller areas such as round the hairline and behind the ears; this is a condition called "pitiriasis" and, like many modern hair disorders, can be triggered off by nerves or emotional tension. It will respond to daily treatment with specially prescribed descaling lotion, but it is best to take professional advice from a registered trichologist (scalp specialist).

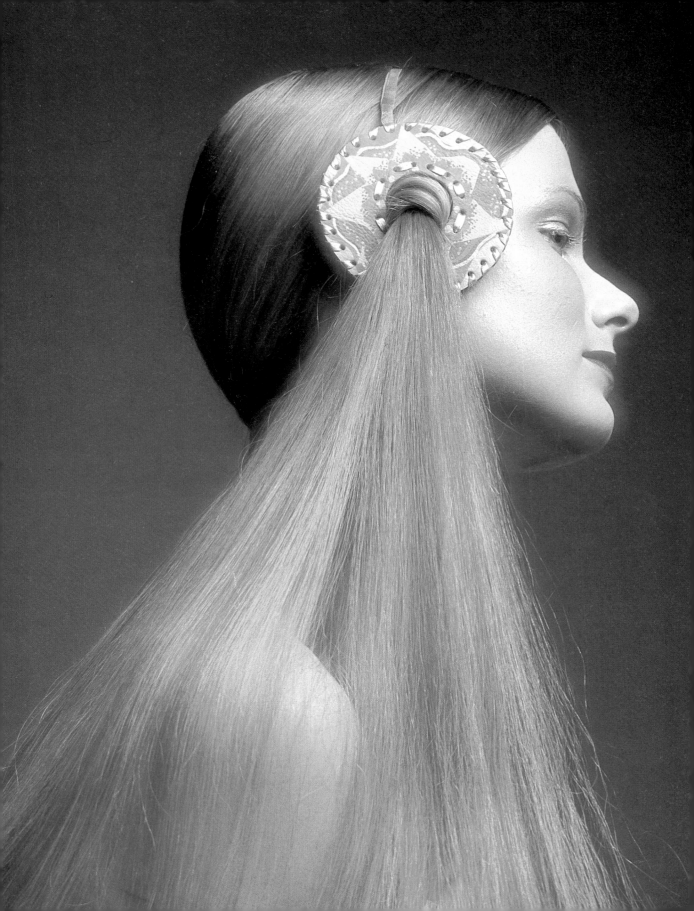

HAIR COLOURING

Modern hair colourants have improved enormously in the last twenty years In the 1920s it was only possible to bleach or henna your hair, and the introduction of natural colours such as all shades of brown, soft gold, and highlighting, is relatively new. The cinema was the first medium to popularize the idea of altering the colour of hair, and blond bombshells such as Jean Harlow did more to promote hair bleaching than anything else did.

Peroxide was the main ingredient of the early bleaches, but this had the disadvantage that if it was used in a mild strength the hair went yellow, while a very strong solution had disastrous effects on the condition of the hair, making it dry and brittle. The cleverness of modern colourants is that they can achieve a natural-looking result without spoiling the texture.

The biggest demand in the hair colour market has always been for a product that covers grey hair and restores it to its natural-looking light, medium or dark brown tones. The colourants of the thirties and forties merely put colour on the outside of the hair, which washed out whenever you shampooed your hair. To overcome this it was necessary to find a way of introducing colour into the hair, and to do this a mild bleaching agent or "para" had to be incorporated into the product. By using this ingredient the colour stayed in the hair for several shampoos and it was possible to colour even white hair so that it blended in and looked completely natural. Many women today use these so-called permanent hair colourants themselves at home, and achieve very successful results.

The main difference between having your colour done professionally and doing it yourself is that a professional colourist will sometimes use a highlighting technique to achieve a more natural light and shade effect.

HIGHLIGHTING

Highlighting, when well done, can be one of the most attractive touches you can add to your hair's appearance. It can look nice on women of any age. But it must be well done, and that in my view means having it done professionally. It is expensive, but nothing looks worse or more ageing than badly done highlighting.

There are two main methods of highlighting hair and both can only be done effectively by a professional colourist. One way is to put a plastic cap on the head and to pull out individual strands for bleaching. The other, and in my opinion the most successful method, is to select very fine strands of hair in layers, apply bleach to them, and then wrap them in foil.

Highlighting can be one of the most attractive effects achieved by modern hairdressing, but it is a real test of a good hairdresser. Badly done it can be a disaster. This striking multi-colour version by Leonard has been achieved using natural herbal colour rinses such as saffron, indigo and henna which give the rainbow effect. These temporary colour rinses are an ideal way of achieving a dramatic effect for a party which will then wash out the next day, leaving you with just your highlights. Modern highlighting techniques give an attractive contrast of light and shade that makes hair look as if it has been lightened by the sun and is very flattering.

A hair ornament like the clasp in this picture by Pablo & Delia can add glamour for a party style.

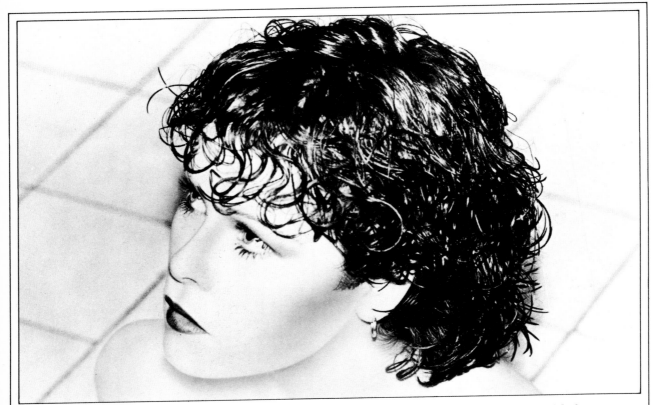

There was a time when if permed hair got wet, it went frizzy and was impossible to control. Modern perms have changed all that. Because of a softer curl, this perm by L'Oréal even looks good after swimming.

PERMS

In this era of natural-looking hair, when a tight set-looking compact style looks so dated, you may think that perms are out of fashion. But perms are very much with us, the difference nowadays being that most perms are not set afterwards. They are an invaluable way of giving body and bounce to straight hair, in fact so much so that men have been having them too. Most of those overall curly styles you see around at present on men owe something to a perm.

As I said earlier, there is no way that any form of conditioning can alter basic hair type, but perming will transform fine straight hair into wavy hair by altering the basic molecular structure of the hair. In the early 1920s, it was discovered that intensive heat applied to the hair when it was tightly wound on to curlers altered the structure of the hair so that it took on a lasting kinkiness. Pictures of pre-war perming methods show ladies strung up to elaborate overhead machines by electric wires which conducted intensive heat to hair that had been wound on

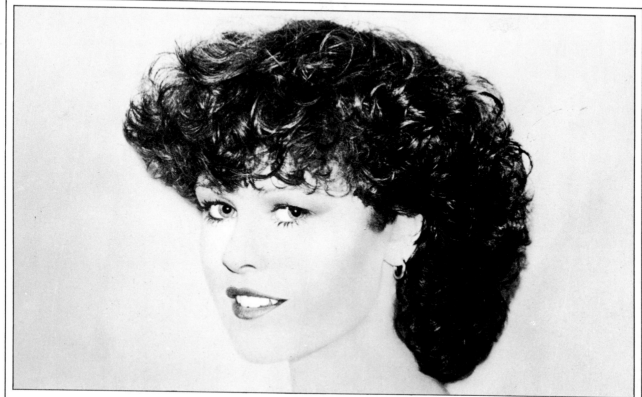

The same perm as seen opposite, but this time it has been blow-dried. These modern soft perms are much easier to manage and don't need to be set on rollers. Joseph Kendall of York Street cut and styled the hair.

small rods. Apart from being very uncomfortable and time consuming, there were many cases of severe scalp burns; the whole process was only feasible because in those days labour was the cheapest part of hairdressing.

Just before the Second World War, however, an American toiletries firm produced a cold wave solution which drastically softened hair so that it could be reshaped to take on the kinky formation of perm curlers. This solution was a derivation of the chemical which had been used successfully to remove superfluous hair on legs. No heat was

required and the advantages of cold permanent waving soon became obvious. Major manufacturers such as Gillette (remember the Toni twins – "which twin has the Toni?"), Unilever and William R. Warner, moved in to market this permanent method for home users.

In the hands of a skilled operator a home perm can be successful. However, bearing in mind the strong properties of the solution – the hair is so softened that it will stretch to three times its normal length without breaking – I feel that it is advisable to go to a professional hairdresser.

The skill in a good perm is not so much in the winding up, although obviously it takes practice to do this quickly, but at the neutralizing stage, which restores hair to its normal elasticity. If your hair is naturally straight, I would strongly recommend having a perm every six months. I find my hair is very much easier to control if I follow this routine.

One of the interesting features of perming and colouring is the tremendous advances that have been made by the leading toiletry firms – mainly continental – in the formulation of products.

In these days when labour is the most expensive part of hairdressing, it has become more and more important that products should be quick and easy to use and completely fool-proof. The days when a hairdresser could afford to buy any old cheap colourant or perm solution from a wholesaler and rely on the skills of his staff to turn out a really well-tinted or permed head of hair have gone. Nowadays most salons prefer to rely on the skills and products of the big hair accessory companies in order to get the best results.

HAIRSTYLES AND MAKE-UP

It does not always occur to women that when they change their hairstyle they may need to alter their make-up. Although hairstyles change more frequently than make-up, they can influence the make-up you wear.

For instance, in the last few years we have had a complete revival of perming which has led to the freaked out "coup sauvage" hairstyles where the hair is left frizzy and unset – in fact the Afro Look. The interesting point about this fashion is that anyone who has tried to wear it with a normal light make-up finds that she looks very plain, and yet when worn with a strongly made-up face the effect is often terrific. For almost the first time I can remember, with the many and varied style changes of the last forty years – ranging from sleek pageboy and upswept bouffant dos, flicked-out bobs, layered urchin cuts, non-styled straight hair and the many versions of the geometric hairstyle – this modern permed style has emphasized the fact that most hard-to-wear hairstyles do rely on a very strong make-up and plenty of emphasis on eyes to give balance to the whole effect.

Another important occasion when you must reconsider whether your make-up suits your hair is when you alter your hair colour. Nothing looks worse than bleached blond hair with too pale a make-up. The skin looks sallow and you tend to look washed out and tired. Lightened hair calls for a warmer make-up with a golden beige or even a pinky beige tone, which is

Coloured hair in brilliant, exotic fantasy shades such as vivid magenta and royal blue may not be most people's idea of a style for them. These two styles created by London's top hairdresser Leonard owe something to modern punk, which has introduced a whole range of fantasy colours. But even if you don't feel like going this far, hair colour can be a valuable addition to many women's looks. The great advances made in the last thirty years in hair colourants have meant that not only can these dramatic colours on the opposite page be achieved, but very natural shades can be available to everyone; the effects can be so natural-looking that it is often impossible to tell whether hair colour has been used.

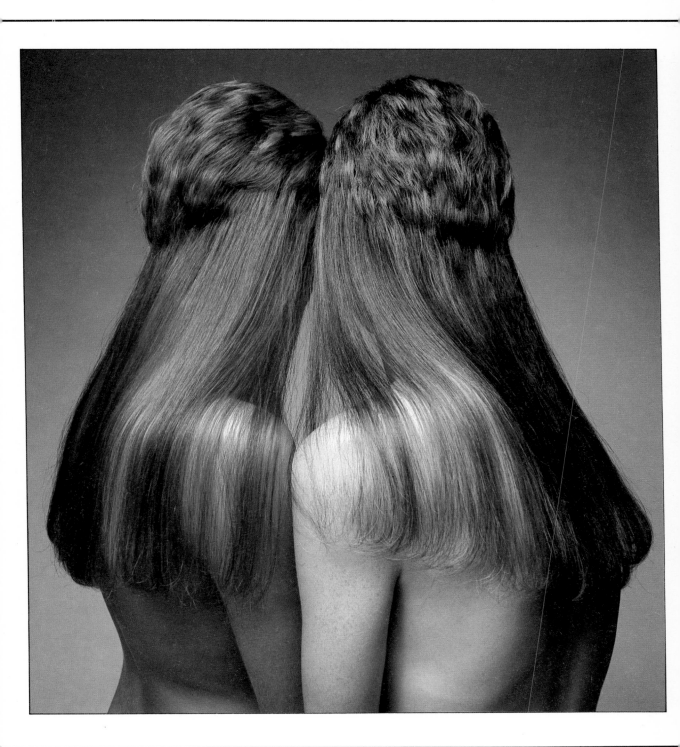

usually much more flattering for lighter hair. This point also applies to people whose hair is going grey. In this case it is necessary to choose a livelier-looking skin tone by warming up your foundation and wearing more blusher. A customer of mine, with lightened hair and a very fair skin, bought an ivory pale foundation and then complained that her skin looked yellow, so she had to change to a warmer pink-toned make-up. However, a few months later she told me that she had gone back to using the pale foundation – because she found that it had suddenly stopped looking yellow for some reason she could not understand and suited her skin again. I noticed that her hair was now several shades darker and this was the reason.

If you are changing the colour of your hair, do not forget your eyebrows will need attention. Nothing looks harder and is a bigger give-away than dark brunette eyebrows with platinum blond hair or even auburn-tinted hair. Ask your hairdresser or your beautician to advise you on what colour your brows should be; they can be toned in to suit your new hair colour with the same tints and lighteners that are used on your hair.

If you are going lighter, remember that your eyebrows may well need thinning, as although thick brows may be consistent with dark hair, they are not very appropriate with lighter hair.

HOME AIDS

The big growth in the "do it yourself" hair market has involved heated rollers, blow-wave combs, portable hair dryers and electric curling tongs: this has meant a change in the pattern of women's hairdressing habits. Leonard says, "We welcome the gadgets, they have all helped to make clients more hair conscious and more prepared to listen to the advice of experts." He also says, quite rightly, that it is mainly because we do not use our heated rollers and other gadgets as well as a professional, that we still have to go to a hairdresser when we want to look our best.

The most useful of all hair aids in my experience are heated rollers. I should be lost without mine. Like so many really useful ideas, the basic idea of a heated roller is remarkably simple. They were invented by a Dane, who patented the idea of filling the curlers with wax and then heating them with an electrical current.

The clever invention of heated rollers first came on to the market in the early 1960s, and Carmen Curlers held the patent on the wax filling which held the heat in the roller curler. Although many manufacturers tried to copy the idea with other heat-retaining substitutes, the Carmen kits are still the most satisfactory of all the heated rollers. As someone who uses them a lot, I find that it is important to use them in conjunction with a conditioning protein setting agent, not an alcohol setting lotion as this would be much too drying. It is only really possible to get a satisfactory result when your hair is well shaped with a professional cut.

The great pitfall of home-styling methods as one gets older is to remember that the excessive tidiness of a set-looking style can be ageing. Ever since the days when lacquered, teased and back-combed hair went out of fashion we have discovered that hair looks prettier and softer when it is not too formally arranged. An interesting feature of the current trend for braided hair is that the hair is dressed in an intricate-looking way which is marvellous for a formal evening occasion, but does not rely for its effect on lacquer and an over-elaborate setting.

As most of the home gadgets involve the use of heat, either to curl or to straighten the hair, conditioning is an important counteraction to the drying effects which make the hair brittle. Currently one of the favourite conditioners is henna, and people who use it regularly swear to its effectiveness and say there is nothing like it for taming "difficult" hair. Made from powdered leaves of Egyptian privet which are mixed with boiling water to a paste, it has traditionally been a colourant and for thousands of years has been used as a natural vegetable dye which brings out the red tones in the hair.

Modern cosmetic chemists have now found that henna also contains effective natural conditioning properties and have produced a non-colouring conditioning wax. The neutral henna used for this wax is made from the leaves of older bushes that have lost their hair-colouring properties but still retain their natural organic conditioners.

Looking after your hair may seem to take a lot of time and sometimes a good deal of money, but it is one of the most critical parts of looking good. Not only can your physical appearance be improved by well-styled healthy hair – most women cannot feel their best unless they know their hair is looking great.

TOTAL BEAUTY

Some people might think that exercise and diet do not fit naturally into a book about make-up. But they do very much. There is little point in having a beautiful face if your body and the way you move do not go some way to complementing it. A good figure is a basic essential of looking good. I believe it is within the reach of most of us if we are prepared to take sufficient trouble, and in my opinion nothing makes you appear younger, particularly as you grow older, than moving with suppleness and grace.

This chapter is not a comprehensive guide to exercising or dieting. There are already many good ones available. What I have attempted to do in this chapter is to give you some personal views on these two subjects and to generate, I hope, in your mind some new ideas about two subjects which I believe are important to our well-being.

EXERCISE

There is one great advantage about living in the current age. We know infinitely more today than our grandmothers did about the beneficial effect of taking exercise. Anyone in her fifties is amazed if she remembers how much older her grandmother looked when she was the same age. Less servants to help us, the more active lives we lead today, and the wearing of shorter skirts and trousers have all made us more mobile.

Many of us were probably put off exercise at school by being made to do PT by an instructor who expected us to do the same exercises as recruits in the army. I well remember being laughed at because I could not climb a rope, always fell off the parallel bars and got stuck on the vaulting horse! The instructors knew their exercises, but did not know which ones were good for young girls, or why they were teaching them.

Let me try to tell you why exercise is so important for all of us. Despite

Practising what she preaches, Joan Price is caught here by Pat Booth doing a yoga headstand. "I practise yoga regularly and, since taking it up fifteen years ago, I find it helps to keep my body flexible and the aches and pains away. One of my favourite pastimes is watching TV standing on my head!"

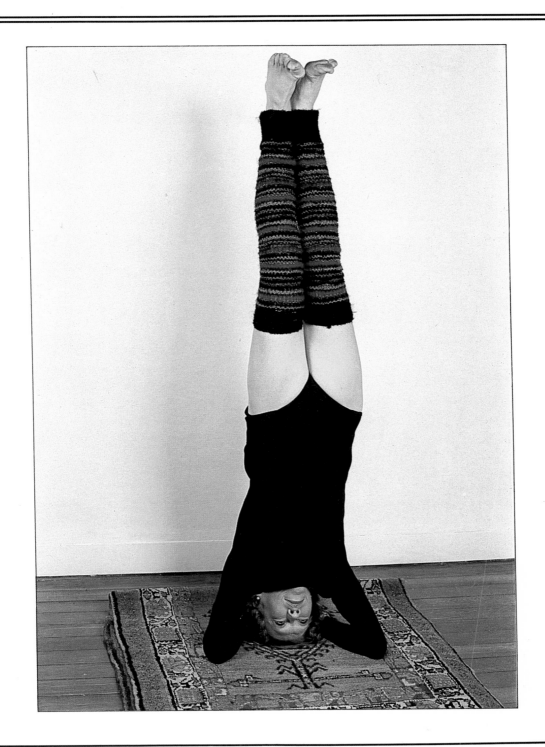

my bad beginning, I realize only too well that if I do not exercise my body gets stiffer and I begin to feel minor aches and pains.

The human body, like the animal body, is built for movement. Although we move around more than our grandparents did, there are still certain aspects of our lives which prevent us from using our bodies naturally. For instance, it is not surprising that so many men and women today suffer from bad backs, considering how much time we spend in cars, sleeping on soft beds and carrying heavy loads. People often say to me, "I lead such an active life that I don't really need to go to exercise classes." But they do not realize the extent to which they under-use their muscles. If you feel this applies to you, it is worth going to an exercise class just to discover how many aches and pains you notice the following day. This can be a salutary experience, especially when you realize that every twinge comes from a muscle which has been completely neglected or under-used and has become slack and out of condition. So often in our daily lives we tend to use the same sets of muscles while neglecting others, such as the stomach muscles which can do so much to support and strengthen our backs.

I have already referred to back problems: let me tell you of two women who have become leading exercise teachers. Both broke their backs and were told that they would never walk again. Through various means both came to realize that one of the keys to a strong back is not the backbone but rather the muscles. It is the muscles in the back which keep the verte-brae in position. Through sheer determination and knowing what to do, these women set about building up their muscles to such a pitch that they provided the broken bones with enough support to heal. One of the women is Joanna Lewis, a leading exponent of the Mensendieck system. The other is a Yoga teacher, and she claims that the non-violent traction which is the feature of this method – you exercise muscles by holding the classic positions or *asanas*, rather than by movement – produced dramatically beneficial results.

I have always been a little sceptical about the value of doctors' advice about bad backs. I feel they are inclined to approach the problem from the bone point of view, relying too much on rest and pain killers, and do not take enough account of the basic cause of the problem, which is so fre-quently weak muscles. So as you will certainly have realized by now, I am a great believer in the value of exercise. But the type of exercise you should do depends very much on the type of person you are, how old you are, how much exercising you have done in the past, and the type of life you lead.

All experts on the back stress how much harm driving in cars, lounging in front of TV, and soft beds do to your back. I am not suggesting that you do not drive, or that you give up watching TV, but I do recommend that when you watch TV you sit in an upright chair, or better still – if the idea is not too revolutionary – on the floor. This is, of course, the Japanese custom, and is particularly good for strengthening your back muscles. Even sitting can be a back exerciser: sit up against a wall with back straight and legs out in front of you, trying not to rely on the wall for support, and you will find that your back muscles will hold you upright for longer and longer periods without sagging. I have practised it for years. Soft beds are certainly not sensible, and worst of all are those beds which sink in at the centre. An increasing number of doctors and physiotherapists recommend that you sleep with a board under your mattress.

Hardly anything can reveal your age as much as the way you move and stand. I often look at women who have spent a great deal of money on face lifts and yet can tell at a glance that they are over fifty, because of the way they walk. A woman of fifty can take ten years off her age if she moves well. And remember that as we get older, our muscles begin to contract and become weaker, and our joints less flexible.

A good starting point to exercise is to walk as much as possible every day, and in particular walk up and down stairs rather than taking the lift. We tend to forget what sedentary lives we lead, making us less mobile and supple. It has always been my observation that the most energetic women I know have remained the youngest in appearance as they have grown old. Exercise also improves breathing and circulation.

I have always found that exercising at home on one's own is not easy, and unless one is talking of a few specific exercises to be done every day to correct, say, weak muscles in the back, I would recommend attending a weekly exercise class. First, this imposes a valuable discipline on you by having to attend regularly; second, if you are going to start exercising, it is sensible to be shown how to do it properly.

There are many different techniques of exercising: all of them have their own advantages and some their disadvantages, but every woman ought to be able to find at least one of these techniques that suits her purposes. In general I am more in favour of the less violent methods, but each of us has her own priorities. But remember, you do not have to be an athletic star or a great games player to exercise: many of the best exponents of Yoga, for instance, are frequently unathletic people. We are not talking about vaulting over wooden horses or similar gymnastic skills. We are talking about suppleness, which is a very different matter to strength.

Overleaf are a few exercises which may be fitted into your daily life.

Loosening Neck and Shoulders

Drop head forward and very slowly rotate to the left as far as your shoulder, then to the right as far as the other shoulder.

Do not go right the way round at the beginning, as you may make yourself feel giddy. After repeating six times, allow the weight of the head to carry you round in a full circle, but do not force it. Repeat this several times.

Lift arms to shoulder level with hands pointing upwards. Rotate arms at shoulder level, backwards and forwards. Repeat ten times both ways.

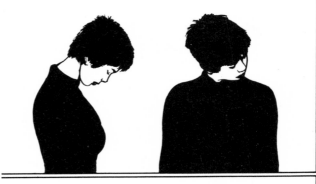

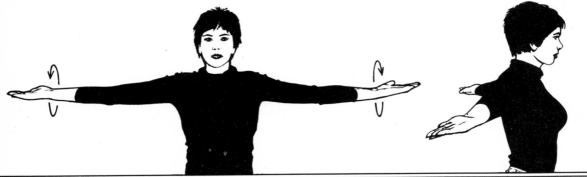

To Tone Upper Arm

Put the back of your left hand as high up between your shoulder-blades as you can, stretch the right arm up above your head, bend the elbow and try to grasp your left hand with your right, behind your shoulders. Hold for a few seconds, and repeat the other side.

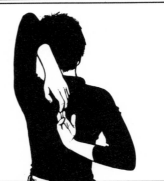

To Firm the Bust

Grasp your wrists in front of you and squeeze hard for a count of five, then relax. Repeat several times.

Put your hands together in front of you, as if you were praying, keeping elbows up. Press palms together hard and hold for a count of ten. Relax and repeat.

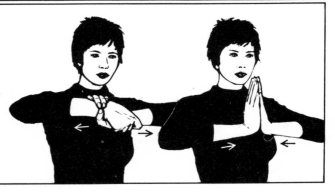

Stomach Improvers

Sit in a chair with your bottom on the front edge, and leaning backwards stretch out your legs in front of you. Lift feet together one inch from the ground and hold for a count of ten. Relax and repeat several times. Keeping the same position do a bicycling movement with the legs.

Stand with legs straight, feet apart, hands on knees. Press down and pull in stomach to try to touch your backbone. Hold for a count of ten, then repeat several times.

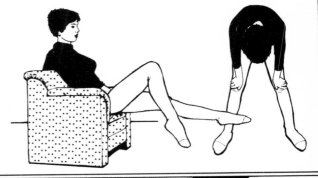

Bottom Toner

Hold on to the back of a chair and press your thighs against it. Lift your left leg to the side, keeping it straight, and swing it across behind you – do not let the thighs move from the chair – hold for a count of ten, then repeat with the right leg.

Stay in the same position and raise leg to the side keeping it straight with the foot turned up. Rotate several times. Repeat with the other leg.

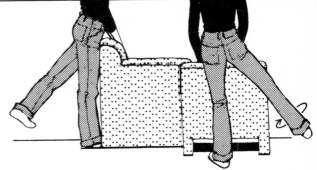

For Tired Legs and Feet

Stand with heels firmly on the ground and bend knees as far as you can without raising the heels. Hold for a few seconds and straighten up – repeat twelve times.

Sit on chair, cross one leg over the other and rotate the foot ten times to the left and ten times to the right. Repeat with the other leg.

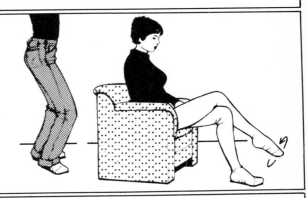

To Firm the Legs

Sit on chair, with legs straight out in front of you and a large book between the feet. Squeeze the book as hard as you can, as if you were trying to bring the legs together. You will feel the leg muscles tightening, and know that this isometric-type exercise is doing you good.

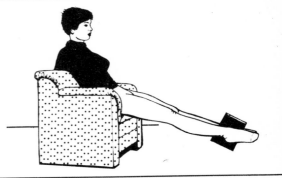

No discussion of the place of exercise in our daily lives would be complete without a reference to jogging. I am not a jogging fan, but there is something to be said in its favour. I have met many Americans who, having discovered my involvement in beauty, almost invariably tell me how much they owe to jogging. They say that since they have taken up jogging, they breathe more easily, feel more relaxed and sleep better.

What jogging basically does is to develop and keep working your heart muscles. Like all the other muscles of your body, these are normally under-used and become flabby and sleepy.

My reservations about jogging are that first, if you are going to do it, you must do it regularly, in fact every day. Second, joggers tend to concentrate just on their heart muscles, to the detriment of the rest of their muscles.

If you are going to take up jogging, remember that it is essential to start off very gently. In no way are you involved in a race with yourself or any-one else. Jogging is only valuable if you do not put a strain on yourself.

SENSIBLE EATING

Few people in this country realize what an important part food plays in their life: it affects both the way you look and the way you feel. In fact, as a generalization, most traditional English eating habits are not very healthy. We tend to rely too much on the frying pan (fish and chips) and starchy puddings, and too little on salads and raw vegetables. The main reasons for taking an interest in and controlling what you eat are, first, that a good diet does help you feel healthier, and second, that overweight is almost invariably due to over eating.

Let me start with the health aspect. I am not a health food fanatic, but I do believe that a good diet is important to general well-being. There is evidence that eating the wrong foods can cause the build-up of toxic waste in the body, which can be related to very serious illnesses. I quote the story of the son of a friend of mine, who was very seriously ill for a number of years, until in desperation his parents took him to a Swedish nutritional expert. He did nothing but alter his eating habits, banning meat and a number of other foods, and switching him to fruit, vegetables, nuts and wholemeal wheat, since when he has been fit and healthy.

I believe that we are only beginning to realize what a difference food can make to the way we feel and look. Just to take the most obvious example of all, anyone who is inclined to spots will find that her skin improves con-siderably if she cuts down on fats and acid-forming carbohydrates and shell fish. That is why I believe that everyone, regardless of whether she is over-weight or not, should take an interest in the food she eats.

The medical profession and dieticians are only beginning to understand fully the important part played by bran in our bread and by cellulose in our vegetables and fruits in keeping us slim. Some medical researchers are beginning to link obesity with the consumption, over many years, of food from which the natural dietary fibre has been removed. Researchers have found that in societies in some parts of Africa, where unrefined foods comprise the main diet, obesity is rare: but once modern civilization arrives with our processed refined foods, obesity starts to develop on a wide scale.

The problem appears to be that some chemical additives used in food processing destroy the vitamins, enzymes and other nutrients in natural foods. This is why it is so important to ensure that your daily diet does contain its share of wholegrain products such as wholewheat bread, brown rice and fresh fruit and vegetables.

There are three basic guidelines to sensible eating:

Eat Regularly and Avoid Snacks
It is important to eat proper meals regularly and not to eat between meals. Snack eating is death to sensible diet: not only does it usually mean that you eat much more than you think, but it almost certainly means that you are eating the wrong type of food. Most snacks tend to have a high carbo-hydrate content and are surprisingly often made from refined sugar and refined flour.

Almost all nutritional experts stress the importance of a good breakfast, preferably high in protein foods like fish, meat, milk and eggs, and it is also better to eat your main meal in the middle of the day rather than in the evening. The reason for this is that at the beginning and middle of the day you are more likely to be energetic after a meal so that the calories consumed during the meal will be used up by the body in exercise.

Eat in Moderation
This is the most difficult of all the eating disciplines. There is ample evidence to show that overweight is caused by over eating, which is why it is so important to understand the principles of sensible eating. The basic requirement of a sensible diet is to eat foods with the right calorific value, in other words, to balance the number of calories you eat every day with the amount of energy you expend. Calories are, after all, only a measure of the energy value of the food that you eat; therefore if you lead a relatively sedentary

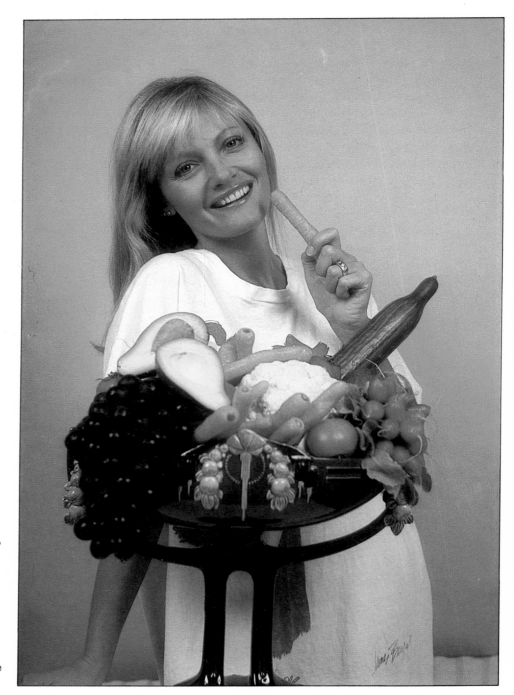

As an example to us all, Pat Booth is photographed by her assistant Andy eating the healthy diet. A former top model, who is married to a doctor, Pat is a strong believer that eating the right foods is important to the way you look.

life you will need to eat less calories than someone who is very active and burning up calories with plenty of energy.

Eat the Right Foods

First and foremost, sensible eating means eating foods that will improve your looks. The old saying "we are what we eat" is true to a certain extent and there is no doubt there are foods which will help to promote strong nails and teeth, healthy hair and skin, and there are rubbish foods which although delicious to eat are actually bad for our looks. Apart from the fact that the latter are the type of foods which put on weight, they also contribute to a build-up of toxic impurities in the system which, even if you are not generally overweight, can produce conditions such as cellulite, that is lumpy-looking fat and lumpy-looking fluid retention on the hips and thighs of women and on the stomachs of men.

The main culprits of rubbish foods are refined sugar and white flour. Most people excuse their craving for sugar by saying they must have it to give them energy; while it is true that it boosts the blood's sugar content to give you instant energy, afterwards it has a let-down effect which can make you feel very slack and tired. With white flour it is ironic that many of us, and this includes myself, eat delicious white crusty bread and then have bran for breakfast – the very ingredient that is removed from the flour in order to make it taste so good. Unless you do eat a certain amount of rough cereal your body and bowels will not function properly.

The important ingredients in a well-balanced diet are protein, fats, and a proportion of carbohydrate. Protein is supplied by fish, poultry, eggs, meat and cheese; fats come mainly from dairy produce and everyone should have half a pint of milk a day as it is a good source of calcium and mineral salts. Because we are all so diet-conscious, many people tend to think that all carbohydrates are bad and identify them with cakes, buns, pastries and chocolates. In fact, carbohydrates include all the fruits and vegetables that you eat, which are so important in providing the body with vitamins and the right proportions of mineral salts, sodium, calcium, potassium and iron, which we need for our general health.

Because cooking can take so much of the goodness out of what we eat, and because many convenience foods lack important vitamins and roughage, a raw salad meal every day is not only better for your figure, but better for your skin, hair, teeth and nails as well.

Most people are unaware of the important part that water plays in sensible eating. Not only does it eliminate waste through the digestive system, but also through the skin by perspiration. It is not generally realized that carbohydrate foods encourage the retention of liquid in the body. If you find you have water retention, the answer is not to cut down on your water intake, but rather to increase it; instead you should cut down on your carbohydrate intake. We should all drink the equivalent of six to eight glasses of liquid a day – not all in tea or coffee with their in-built stimulants. Glasses of plain water are best.

If you do not drink sufficient liquid, you will find that you do not perspire sufficiently and you will retain too much toxic waste. Perspiration is an important way for the body to rid itself of impurities. Many diets recommend that you start the day by drinking a glass of warm water with the juice of a lemon.

This brings me on to the subject of alcohol. There is little doubt in my mind that alcohol in moderation is a valuable social lubricant and helps us to relax. The problem is that there is no question that all alcohol is fattening, as sugar is the basis of fermentation.

If you are trying to lose weight, it is best to try to give up drinking alcohol for a time, but very few people wish to adopt this as a permanent way of life. My advice is to try to limit alcohol to social occasions; that dry white wine has the lowest calorie count; and that mixers such as bitter lemon and tonic are almost as fattening as the alcohol itself, unless you confine yourself to the slimline varieties. It is also sensible to limit yourself to as narrow a range of drinks as possible.

Dieting to Lose Weight

So much is talked and written about this subject that people tend to get confused. If you think you need to slim you should check with your doctor first. Although you will always find someone who swears by a particular diet, it is important to realize that there are no miracle diets and if a friend has found an answer that seems to suit her particular requirements, it is unlikely that the same eating programme will work as well for you.

There is currently a certain amount of discussion about whether doctors and the medical profession are putting too much emphasis on the need to slim. There is a view that overweight people should be encouraged to come to terms with their weight and should not be frightened and worried into losing weight. I do not intend to get involved in the medical pros and cons of overweight. This is a beauty book, and is about how to make the best of yourself, and as far as that is concerned there is no way that overweight is going to be any help whatsoever. I should add also that I have always been struck at the excitement that successful Weight Watchers have felt at getting themselves back to normal weight. It has been intriguing to see the sudden new interest that the women slimmers have taken in making the most of their appearance.

Virtually every dietary expert is now agreed that overweight is caused by over eating, though incidentally over eating does not always cause overweight. There are some people whose metabolism burns up their calories so quickly that more or less regardless of what they eat, they never get fatter; but there are not that many lucky people!

Fat people always find it hard to accept that they eat more than other people. To a large extent over eating is a matter of habit. Frequently it has to do with upbringing. If you come from a family which is used to having large helpings, or always a second helping, you may not realize that what you consider to be a normal helping is probably fifty per cent more than most other people are used to.

I have mentioned in an earlier chapter that I have judged Weight Watchers Competitions for Bernice Weston. Seeing and talking to men and women who have weighed over eighteen stone and have reduced themselves to normal sizes has persuaded me it is what you eat and how much that affect your weight.

Unlike the articles you read in newspapers and magazines, virtually every nutritional expert is unanimous in their condemnation of "gimmicky diets". You may well ask, "Why do so many newspapers carry such articles?" The reason, I am afraid to say, is that editors, who have seldom bothered to enquire into nutritional questions, feel that these diets are more newsworthy and exciting to the readers.

Having said that, there are a few points in favour of crash diets: diets such as bananas and milk, consommé and cottage cheese, fruit and yoghurt, or any combination of low-fat foods are easy to prepare and will give you a quick weight loss in the shortest possible time. The problem with such diets is that they cannot be a way of life, and are short-term solutions. But at least having done it once you know that the next time you can lose weight if you want to; it also means that you are at least aware that you have a weight problem. But most nutritional experts are agreed that if you are overweight, you must attack the problem by understanding that you need to alter your eating habits for life. Losing weight is only the beginning of solving the problem: keeping your weight down is a much greater test of stamina and character.

There are basically two ways of controlling your diet long term. One is to go on a carbohydrate counting system, and the other is to count your calories. Counting only your carbohydrates became popular with the publication of the "drinking man's diet". This system restricts your intake of carbohydrate foods drastically; not only the sugar and starch foods, but also vegetables and fruit. Drink was also included on the carbohydrate list. Non-carbohydrate foods such as meat, chicken, fish, cheese and eggs are listed as free foods. I have known people adopt this diet who have found that because they only have to count certain categories of foods it has been more successful than a calorie-controlled diet where you have to count the value of everything you eat. I think the weakness of the carbohydrate-controlled diet is that a too high protein diet is not good for everyone, and also you need more self-control for this type of diet to be successful simply because of the "unrestricted food category" which means that you are inclined to eat some foods, such as cheese, too freely.

Calorie-controlled diets are the basis of nearly all the regimes that you find in magazines and newspapers, where the dietary expert has selected a theme for a diet, and then put it together keeping the overall count down to a limited number of calories. It is probably the most satisfactory method that has been found for measuring the amount of food that the body needs to keep it healthy yet not overweight. The number of calories in a particular food is an accurate guide to its fattening power. By consuming less calories than you need each day you are bound to lose weight. It is important to remember, once you have decided to follow one system or the other, to get yourself a good calorie counter guide or carbohydrate counter and free food list. But it is definitely not advisable to try to follow both systems at the same time.

Most dieticians recommend that when dieting a man should cut his calorie count down to 1500 a day and a woman to 1200. Once you have established the weight you wish to remain at, the average man needs about 3000 calories a day, and a woman about 1900.

I am certain that this straightforward and disciplined way of counting calories is the most sensible way of dieting, as it means that you are facing the problem head-on. This brings me to the subject of "slimming foods", about which I believe there are a number of misconceptions. Most dieticians will tell you that it is better to stick to normal foods in smaller quantities, rather than rely on cutting your calories by eating low calorie substitutes. This is partly because you are not always eating at home, and partly because discipline is basically the answer to all slimming and there are no easy answers. I have far fewer reservations about low calorie drinks, which fulfil a useful social role.

When talking to audiences about sensible eating, I usually add a few special points as guidance:

DON'T spend too much time studying menus in restaurants: one of the biggest threats to any careful eater's good resolutions is a menu: try and decide what you will eat *before* you look at any tempting recommendations

DON'T weigh yourself too often: constant weight checks on different scales can show too much fluctuation: weigh yourself once a week at the same time of day

DON'T hold an empty glass at a party: keep it filled with low calorie tonic, bitter lemon or tomato juice

DON'T listen to well-meaning friends: comments like "I think a bit of weight suits you", "Go on, one slice of cake won't hurt you", can be well meaning but dreadful saboteurs

DO face the naked truth in front of a mirror: friends may tell you you are not overweight, but only you can really decide by standing in front of a full-length mirror without clothes to hide the bulges

DO banish the frying pan: foods should be grilled or steamed rather than fried

DO be prepared for failure: do not be too easily discouraged – all right, so you really broke all the rules yesterday, but that does not mean that you are giving up your sensible eating plan for ever

DO accept that medications like the contraceptive pill can have an adverse effect on your weight: it can happen and it may be the particular pill you are taking: if in doubt consult a doctor

Incidentally, do not think that slimming or low calorie foods are of value as part of your normal diet. If you are going to use them, they only really work if you stick to a fairly rigid daily calorie count.

One of the major problems for many women in trying to slim is how to do it when you have to cook and feed a growing family. Judging from friends and acquaintances who have slimmed, you need to have enormous self-discipline to do it on your own without any help. Most of the people I know who have managed to slim successfully have joined a slimming club.

There is no doubt that the mutual help and encouragement that you get from other slimmers is an advantage. It does not mean if you join one of these clubs that you are bound to lose weight, but I think you have a better chance of persevering with the battle.

Before finishing this chapter, I must mention the "fluid diet". It is a system practised by many health hydros and is basically not a slimming diet, but more important it allows the body to de-coke and rid itself of its impurities. Some exponents have a regular "fluid-only" day on fruit juice, consomme, and herb tisanes, say once a month; some even do it once a week, and I cannot think of a better way of pointing out what it can do for you than telling you that one of the keenest disciples of a regular weekly de-coke is Katie Boyle, the well-known broadcaster. But whatever you do, do not experiment on a working day. It is a sensible idea to check with your doctor before trying it out for the first time.

Do take note of some of the points that I have made in this final chapter, because however beautiful your face, you are unlikely to feel completely satisfied and at one with yourself unless it is complemented by a beautiful body.

ACKNOWLEDGEMENTS

The authors and publishers would like to express their appreciation to the following for permission to reproduce photographs in *Making Faces*: AP Feature Photos *(picture on page 33)*; David Bailey *(page 37)*; BBC Hulton Picture Library *(pages 24, 25, 26, 60)*; Biba *(page 39)*; Camera Press *(pages 29, 45)*; Cooper-Bridgeman Library *(pages 9, 111)*; Elisabeth Photo Library *(page 20)*; Essanelle *(page 163)*; Eve of Roma *(page 36)*; Harriet Hubbard Ayer *(page 22)*; Barry Latigan *(pages 166, 171)*; Serge Lutens at Christian Dior *(page 62)*; Michael Mann Studio *(page 15)*; The Mansell Collection *(page 13)*; Max Factor *(page 28)*; Mobile Press Photos *(pages 168, 169)*; MW Publicity *(pages 34, 40)*; The National Magazine Company *(page 7)*; Popperfoto *(pages 29, 30, 32, 35, 39, 45)*; Portman Press Bureau Ltd *(page 79)*; Mary Quant Cosmetics Ltd *(page 37)*; Revlon *(pages 31, 139)*; Helena Rubinstein *(page 25)*; Vidal Sassoon *(pages 157, 158)*; Syndication International *(page 60)*; Paul Tanqueray *(page 23)*; John Topham *(page 33)*; United Press International *(page 35)*. Thanks are also due to David Warmington for his illustrations on pages 67, 70, 71, 122, 123, 146, 178 and 179.

INDEX